ABOU ... :E AUTHORS

Kirsten Hartvig was born in Denmark and
studied Herbal Medicine in England at the
School of Herbal Medicine, Tunbridge Wells.
She later completed a post-graduate training in
Naturopathic Medicine at the British College of
Naturopathy and Osteopathy, London. She is a
member of the National Institute of Medical
Herbalists and the Register of Naturopaths.

In addition to her clinical work, Kirsten has
taught Nutrition and Dietetics at the European
School of Osteopathy and now gives regular
lectures on health and nutrition to a variety of
professional and lay groups in Denmark and
Britain. She collaborated with Geoffrey Cannon
on *Superbug* and has written articles
on health and nutrition for various publications.

Dr Nic Rowley read medicine at Trinity
College, Cambridge and completed his clinical
training in London. He is also qualified in accupuncture.
He was Vice-Principal at the European School of
Osteopathy, and has worked as an holisitic physician
in multi-disciplinary practices in Kent and West
Sussex.

Nic is the author of two other books. *Basic
Clinical Science, Describing a Rose with a Ruler* is a
standard reference for students of complementary
medicine. His most recent book is *Hands On, A
Manual of Clinical Skills.*

YOU ARE WHAT YOU EAT

An easy-to-follow naturopathic guide
to good food and better health

KIRSTEN HARTVIG ND
& DR NIC ROWLEY

PIATKUS

This book is dedicated to
Joyce and Clem Thomas,
with love and thanks

© 1996 Kirsten Hartvig and Nic Rowley

First published in 1996 by
Judy Piatkus (Publishers) Limited
5 Windmill Street
London W1P 1HF

First paperback edition 1997

ISBN 0–7499–1591–9 (Hbk)
ISBN 0–7499–1714–8 (Pbk)✓

Designed by Paul Saunders
Diagrams by Rodney Paul

Typeset by Phoenix Photosetting, Lordswood, Chatham, Kent
Printed and bound in Great Britain by Mackays of Chatham PLC

CONTENTS

PREFACE

This book has grown out of our work as health-care practitioners and teachers of nutrition and medical science. Though trained in the art of giving treatments – one of us as a herbalist, naturopath and psychotherapist, the other as an orthodox doctor and acupuncturist – we no longer see patients in formal consultations. Instead we run retreats in which people spend time in peaceful surroundings, paying attention to the basics of life – rest, good food, physical activity, creativity and community. We live and work in this way because our experience of dealing with illness has taught us that nature has an in-built tendency to heal when given the right conditions; and that everyone can increase their self-healing ability by improving the quality of their food.

We owe a debt of gratitude to the many patients, students and colleagues who have taught us so much about food, health and healing and humbly acknowledge the wisdom of those teachers past and present whose ideas are echoed here. In particular we would like to thank Dr Joyce Thomas, Linda Wilkinson, Anna Mews, Geoffrey Cannon, Richard Farhall, Mario Szewiel, Christine Steward, Dr Derek Wolfe, Keith and Maureen Robertson, Lilly Jensen, Dr Joseph Goodman, Tim Coysten, Tessa Hodsdon, Nigel and Amanda Brooke, Anthony Milroy, Holly Regan-Jones, Sara Damskier, Ernst Frederiksen, Frances and Paul Büning Hambly, Pamela Blake-Wilson, Nick Beak, Else Veje, Jeanette Cold and Heather Rocklin for their help, advice and inspiration. Any errors or omissions are, however, our responsibility.

FOREWORD

Kirsten Hartvig and Nic Rowley have written a lovely book. I believe their personal partnership – their being wife and husband – as well as their joint knowledge and wisdom and their intimate relationship as co-authors, gives *You Are What You Eat* a special value. This is a book which has been felt as well as thought through.

There are a number of reasons why anything written by Kirsten and Nic deserves your trust. Both of them understand and respect the peculiar versions of science and medicine now dominant in the industrialised world, but, with respect, they put reductionist science and allopathic medicine in their place as useful tools, subsidiary to the **real** business of understanding health, life, and our purpose here on the planet. They are also both excellent researchers, who as good market gardeners do, enjoy digging for facts, nurturing ideas, and organising information in appetising ways. I don't agree with every single thing they write here, but I advise you to be guided by them.

Most people who pick up this book in a shop and consider buying and using it have more opportunity now to look after themselves and thus a better chance of enjoying a healthy and vigorous long life than people at any other time in history.

Take cancer, for example, a field in which I am currently working. As with heart disease, the rational approach to cancer is prevention. Although cancer has a genetic aspect and although the possibility of cancer increases with age, most cancer has environmental causes. Something like two-thirds of all cancer deaths are preventable by two simple means: not smoking and eating well. What that means is that at least 100,000 deaths a year from cancer in the UK, and 500,000 deaths a year from cancer in the EU, are preventable if, throughout life, people choose to take the avice set out in *You Are What You Eat*.

Or take infectious disease, a field in which Kirsten and I have worked together. As with non-infectious diseases like cancer, the rational approach to infectious disease is naturopathic. This means you need to live well and eat well and, if you are suffering symptoms from some infection, to rest and give the body the best chance to heal and strengthen itself against disease. There is a place for drugs, just as there is a place for surgery, but drugs are usually best used only as a last resort or when life itself is threatened.

And as Kirsten and Nic know, the ancient learning which forms the basis for most of the healing arts all over the world and throughout history, which for a brief strange period in the West has been ignored or even persecuted as witchcraft, is now becoming vindicated by the findings of researchers in the biological sciences. For example, plant-based diets really do protect against cancer. Throughout this century until the 1980s this concept was generally dismissed as a foolish dream. But now, many hundreds of reliable epidemiological and experimental studies show that fresh vegetables, fruits and pulses are stuffed with bioactive compounds, mostly off the map of nutritional science, which are likely to protect against cancer. What they are and why this is nobody yet knows exactly for sure, which, in turn, shows that nature is often best respected, not dissected, and that sometimes knowledge drives out wisdom.

You Are What You Eat is meant to be used. Keep it in the kitchen. Enjoy.

Geoffrey Cannon
Chairman, National Food Alliance

INTRODUCTION

You Are What You Eat is a book about naturopathic nutrition, a fresh approach to healthy eating based on age-old knowledge. It describes how to make any diet healthy by using cheap, widely available foods and without taking vitamin and mineral supplements. It shows how good food protects against the diseases that afflict modern society and explains why eating healthy food makes the environment more healthy. *You Are What You Eat* is about changing the world by choosing what you put in your mouth.

We all eat to live and have basic nutritional needs, but many popular beliefs about nutrition are myths based on prejudiced and out-dated research. As a result, there is confusion about what the nutritional needs of the human being really are, a situation made worse by complex scientific reference books and food composition tables.

You Are What You Eat is an attempt to cut through this confusion by combining simple explanations of natural nutritional principles with clear information about the nutritional content of common foods. It is written for all who are interested in improving health by improving diet and who would like a concise, up-to-date source of nutritional information. It uses the best of traditional and modern dietary knowledge to demystify nutrition and to help you to make informed choices about your food.

Part One describes what naturopathic nutrition is and outlines the basic principles of healthy eating. Part Two explains how to analyse your diet and transform it into a new way of eating that improves your health, increases your energy level and gives you a new sense of well-being. Part Three shows how diet can be used in the treatment of illness and includes information on the healing properties of various common foods. The Appendices provide you with basic information about the nutritional content of food.

The principles of naturopathic nutrition will help you to create a diet rich in essential nutrients. By eating more of what is good for you instead of worrying about what is bad for you, you will eat more complex carbohydrates, fibre, vitamins and minerals and less fat and sugar. By filling your stomach with healthy food, you will leave less room for the unhealthy.

You Are What You Eat is a book that will give you control over your diet and your health. We hope it will help you to get the most out of your life.

PART ONE: FOOD FOR LIFE

CHAPTER ONE

SAGES AND LONE VOICES

Naturopathic ideas are as old as history and have influenced all the great medical traditions of the world. In this chapter, we look at the history of naturopathic thought.

For many thousands of years, the human race has managed to evolve without any technical knowledge of nutrition. In the great ancient healing traditions of Egypt, China, India, Greece and Native America, simple whole foods, herbs, water, fresh air, sunshine and exercise were used to promote and maintain health, and wellness was seen as the natural state. Disease was regarded as an expression of disharmony in a person's life or environment, a disturbance of the balance between body, mind and spirit. When illness came, this balance was restored by a partnership between the healing power of nature and the self-healing ability of the body – a partnership which is called naturopathy.

Hippocrates (460–377BC), the 'Father of Medicine', is naturopathy's best known son. Heir to a philosophy as old as thought itself, he used good food, water, air, exercise, fasting and advice on lifestyle as the basis for treatment of disease. He helped people to reconnect with the source of knowledge of the laws of life and living, because he knew that where health is increased, disease naturally decreases. His most celebrated saying, 'above all, do no harm', is the basic principle of naturopathic nutrition and expresses one of life's fundamental truths – that doing good does good.

Hippocrates believed that Man and Nature were interdependent, and expressed his beliefs in the following laws of health:

1. Only nature heals, provided it is given the opportunity to do so.

2. Let food be your medicine, let medicine be your food.

3. Disease is an expression of purification.

4. All disease is one.

5. It is more important what sort of person has a disease than what sort of disease a person has.

Like Pythagoras before him, Hippocrates was part of an unbroken tradition of naturopathic thought which the Essenes, the Druids, the Cathars and countless others have kept alive ever since. He used methods that were humane, rational and based on respect for each person's individual responsibility for their own health. Like the Welsh Physicians of Myddfai, who passed the simple truths of naturopathic practice down through the ages until the eighteenth century, Hippocrates knew that 'whosoever shall eat or drink more or less than he should, or shall sleep more or less, or shall labour more or less from idleness or from hardship, without doubt he will not escape sickness'.

However, despite the honour still paid to the memory of Hippocrates by the physicians of today, his principles no longer motivate modern medicine. The influence of Galen – a court physician in Rome during the latter part of the second century AD, 500 years after Hippocrates – has had a much greater effect on the development of orthodox medical thinking. The teachings of Galen are important because they were the cornerstones of a non-naturopathic, elaborate and rigid system of medicine that effectively paralyzed European medical thinking for 1500 years. They marked the beginning of the divisions in philosophy and practice which still distinguish the 'modern' physician from the naturopathic doctor.[1]

Galen favoured elaborate, costly medicine consisting of dozens of ingredients. Following his lead, physicians came to believe that the more complex a remedy, the better it was. Prescriptions became stronger, containing exotic substances from the animal and the mineral kingdoms such as viper's flesh, crushed deer antlers, crab's eyes, rhinoceros and unicorn horn, oil of earthworms, powdered mummy, the moss from a dead man's skull and goat's urine. Health and disease became the domain of university graduates, who spent years learning Galen's complex writings (and, later on, Avicenna's) and who had little time for the use of simple foods or wayside weeds in the treatment of disease.

It is interesting that we now believe that it was witches and Druids who used spider's legs and frog's eyes in their medicines. In fact, those remedies were used by orthodox doctors who found a ready market for their

[1] Doctor was the Greek word for 'teacher'.

mysterious preparations in those willing to pay for freedom from responsibility for their own health. Village wise women relied on natural principles
and simple plant remedies and held to the view that each of us is responsible for our own health.

Despite Galen's powerful influence, naturopathic methods remained in
use in various parts of the world. In the ninth century, Rhazes (also known
as Ar-Razi) emphasized the importance of diet and hygiene rather than
drugs, saying that 'where a cure can be obtained by diet, use no drugs and
avoid complex remedies where simple ones will suffice'. In the following
century, Ibn Butlan wrote in the *Taquim as-Sihhah* of the importance of rest,
clean air, moderate diet and 'the evacuation of superfluities'. In his opinion,
if all these were kept in balance, health resulted. When they were out of harmony, sickness occurred.

In the tenth century, a school of natural medicine was founded in the
small south-Italian town of Salerno. It became a centre for the teaching and
practice of Hippocratic medicine based on moderation in diet, sufficient
sleep, fresh air and exercise.

As the Renaissance started to unfold in western Europe, Galen's teachings still ruled the medical establishment. They were strongly challenged
by Paracelsus (1493–1541), however, who believed that natural practices
were far superior to the Galenic medicine of his day, which he missed no
opportunity to attack and ridicule. At heart, Paracelsus was a naturopath
who considered the body to be an integrated whole, with all parts
interacting and communicating with each other and also with the wider
universe outside. However, his fascination for chemistry and alchemy led
him to believe that if the 'active ingredients' of plants could be found,
perfect medicines could be invented; it is for this idea[1] that he is still
remembered.

Galen's authority finally crumbled when, in 1628, William Harvey proved
that – contrary to Galen's teachings – the blood circulated around the body.
Unfortunately, physicians had become so used to working within a rigid
Galenical system by this time that they felt driven to invent a new system
involving bleeding, blistering and strong purgatives as the treatments of
choice for nearly all conditions. The effects of such treatments were often
even more disastrous for patients than Galen's mixtures had been, and the
sick person's lot became ever more hazardous.

Lone voices still spoke up for a more natural approach, however. As
Nicholas Culpepper wrote in the early 1600s, '... I would they [the physi-
cians] would consider what infinite number of poor creatures perish daily

---

[1] An idea still cherished by medical orthodoxy.

who else might happily be preserved if they knew but what the Herbs in their own Garden were good for'.

By the eighteenth century, the relationship between food and disease had been all but forgotten by a medical establishment dependent on bleeding and on highly toxic medicines containing mercury and antimony. But amongst ordinary people, wary of the exotic mixtures offered by the apothecaries, the simple counsel of village wise women and naturopaths like Dr William Buchan remained popular. In 1769, Buchan wrote, 'I think the administration of medicine always doubtful, and often dangerous and would much rather teach men (*sic*) how to avoid the necessity of using them than how they should be used ...' True to his words, he published *Domestic Medicine*, which emphasized the importance of diet, hygiene, cleanliness, simple foods and herbal remedies; the volume sold in thousands.

Even the British Admiralty was obliged to consider the link between health and diet when naval surgeon, James Lind (1716–1794), researching the scourge of scurvy amongst British servicemen, concluded that '... as greens or fresh vegetables with ripe fruits are the best remedies for it, so they prove the most effectual preservative against it'. The Admiralty ordered that every sailor should have lemon juice on long voyages and within two years, scurvy vanished from the British Navy.

In America, despite the astonishing example of the native people's good health, the health-giving potential of good food and local plants was also largely ignored. Most American physicians at the time believed that disease was an enemy to be attacked with the strongest weapons available, and did not believe that nature had a role to play in healing. However, the self-taught naturopath Samuel Thompson (1769–1843) spoke forcefully against the use of poisonous medicine in the New World. At the same time, the German doctor, Samuel Hahnemann (1755–1843), was founding a system of homeopathic medicine based on the body's self-healing ability and nature's healing forces.

By the beginning of the nineteenth century, the excesses of 'bleeding and mercury' medicine were such that even members of the medical establishment were calling for renewed recognition of the healing powers of nature. Many doctors rejected orthodox medicines in favour of 'nature cure', involving 'plenty of exercise, fresh mountain air, water treatments in cool, sparkling brooks and simple, wholesome country fare consisting largely of bread and vegetables'. One prominent university lecturer at the time wrote: 'Whatever elements nature does not introduce in vegetables (the natural food of all animal life – directly of herbivorous, indirectly of carnivorous) are to be regarded with suspicion'. Naturopaths like John Skelton in England, Vincenz Priessnitz in Europe and Henry Lindlahr in America were part of a renaissance of naturopathic thinking. And yet, for the poor and deprived, the new urban industrial age brought even greater poverty accompanied by its constant companion, disease, made worse by the blinkered use of mercury and bleeding by orthodox physicians.

By the end of the 1800s, chemistry – orthodox medicine's long time concubine – had developed out of the smoke of industrial ambition into a powerful science, and the First World War triggered a pharmacological explosion of synthetic drug production. The medical profession began to look forward to a time when artificial drugs would be able to produce any desired effect on the body; scientists worked hard to improve modern 'chemotherapy' and 'to wash away the plant and vegetable debris' of the old medicines.

Nevertheless, until the Second World War and the arrival of antibiotics, health spas remained popular and natural health programmes were much in demand. One such programme, devised by naturopath, Benedict Lust (1869–1945), consisted of 'the elimination of bad habits, the introduction of corrective habits (proper breathing, exercise, mental attitude and moderation) and new principles of living (fasting, wholefoods, light, air baths, mud baths, and osteopathy)'.

Since 1945, however, peace, fresh air, clean water, rest and good nutrition have slowly gone out of fashion again, as a 'quick fix' attitude has infected medical practice and the expectations of patients. Until quite recently, many people still believed it possible to find a 'pill for every ill' and the West seemed to be witnessing 'a chemotherapeutic revolution which reduced nearly all non-viral diseases to the significance of a bad cold', as Dr David Moreau wrote in 1976. He concluded, 'if the competitive drug industry is allowed to continue the extraordinary achievements of the last sixty years, by 2036 nearly all the health obstacles to survival into extreme old age will have been overcome'.

But the Magic Bullets of the 1960s, '70s and '80s were not usually designed to stimulate the body's own natural healing ability; they were often devised to suppress painful symptoms by blocking or suppressing bodily functions. The blocking or suppressive action of modern drugs may remove some of the distressing effects of disease, but often leaves the cause untouched. What is more, adverse reactions as a consequence of drug therapy become ever more troublesome. The chronic disease epidemics of the late twentieth century seem to bear tragic witness to the fact that there really is no such thing as 'a quick fix' when it comes to health.

In many ways, of course, the human race has taken giant steps in understanding natural laws since the time of Hippocrates. It has certainly learnt to extract the things it wants from nature and use them to its advantage. Yet it has forgotten what to do with the things that are left, and the price has been pollution – internal, as well as external.

So now the wheel is turning again. Health spas in Europe and America are beginning to thrive as patients look outside orthodox medicine for help with their ills. Naturopathic ideas are fuelling a renaissance in natural health care as individuals, families and communities start to reclaim responsibility for their own health. More and more people are recognizing that, given the right conditions, the human body has phenomenal self healing power, a power based on our most fundamental energy: vitality.

CHAPTER TWO

YOU ARE WHAT YOU EAT

In this chapter, we look at the concept of vitality and describe the principles of naturopathic nutrition, the oldest, simplest and most effective way of eating for health.

Vitality and the healing power of nature

Vitality is the energy of being alive. It can also be called life force. Vitality makes the heart beat, provides the will to live and keeps the body healthy in a changing world by enabling it to resist damage and carry out its many different functions.

Living beings are made of matter and vitality. Anyone who has seen a dead body knows that this is true, because although a dead body is made of the same substance as a live one, it is obvious that something is missing. Without life force, a body is like a car with the engine turned off, a ship without a crew. Vital energy flows through all living things and is our link to the healing power of nature. It is the flight of an eagle on a thermal wind, soaring effortlessly above the world. It is the power of an acorn containing a giant oak where birds will nest. It is a flower breaking through the tarmac on a hot summer's day. It is everything striving to be and to become, to belong.

When vitality is recognized as the basis of life, health becomes more than just the absence of disease. It is redefined as the life force fully in charge of the body. In health, the life force enables the body to function in harmony with the external environment by creating an harmonious internal environment. It helps body structures to work easily and comfortably without accumulating waste. However, if the life force loses control of organs or tissues, the affected parts become unable to fulfil their duties and we start to look and feel unwell. The more parts that are affected, the less the body is able to meet the challenges of life and the more unwell we become. If all vitality is lost, we die.

Maintaining health is therefore a matter of maintaining vitality, and healing is doing whatever is necessary to reconnect diseased tissues with the life force so that physiological, biochemical, emotional, mental and spiritual harmony can be restored. From this perspective, illness turns into something helpful, not harmful, because it shows us when our vitality is depleted. It offers us a chance to correct the things that decrease our life force before we become seriously unwell; in the long run, it enables us to become healthier and stronger than we were before.

Like plants, when our living conditions are good, our vitality is high. Also like plants, the best way to restore vitality when health declines is to pay attention to the basics of life – sunlight, water, nourishment and comfort. Naturopathic nutrition is about getting the basics right; it is a way of turning food into vitality.

The principles of naturopathic nutrition

Naturopathic nutrition is based on the simple idea that the best approach to life is to encourage the good, rather than to attack the bad. Instead of being at war with 'bad' habits, it suggests concentrating on good habits, because this naturally reduces the space, time and energy given to those things that do us harm. Diets made up of restrictions and prohibitions are often boring and hard to follow. Naturopathic nutrition fills the body with healthy food so that the need for unhealthy food naturally drops away. It works *with* the powerful forces of nature and helps us to use the natural healing power of the life force within us. Naturopathic nutrition helps to ensure that our cells are properly nourished, that repairs are carried out when needed and that waste products are properly dealt with by the body. Like nature, it helps us to make the best use of what we have, instead of being limited by what we are missing.

We are a part of nature, subject to its rules and regulations. Our bodies respond to its rhythms. We are part of an ecological system where the strongest survive, a system in which life constantly changes in response to opposing forces which build things up and break them down. Worms in the soil help to decompose materials that have lost vitality into basic chemical components which are, in turn, absorbed by plants and used to build new life forms. Germs break down weakened organisms and help to ensure that only strong genes are carried forward into new generations. But there is no war between good and evil in nature; every creature and every plant strives for perfection by putting energy into things that *work*, whilst releasing and recycling the energy contained in things that don't. Nature makes things grow out of whatever is available at the time.

Naturopathic nutrition recognizes that if you are alive, then at least *some* things are working properly. When you recognize what is working well and give it more attention and encouragement, vitality is increased and health improves. If, through illness, your body or mind become your opponent, the solution is to praise what is good in your opponent and see it respond by wanting to please you. As in other areas of life, praise is at least as good a tool as criticism, and the quickest way to end an argument is to find something about which to *agree*. It is better to relieve illness by encouraging self-healing, rather than punishing self-healing by suppressing its symptoms and signs.

The object of natural nutrition is to promote and restore health by encouraging the self-healing potential within each person and it achieves this by following one basic principle: you are what you eat.

If you have ever tried filling the tank of a petrol-engined car with diesel fuel, you will know that after a lot of coughing, spluttering and black smoke belching from the exhaust, the engine refuses to work. Of course, diesel fuel is not bad in itself; it is just not good for cars with petrol engines.

In the same way, if we consume foods robbed of their natural qualities by processing, refining, irradiation and chemical adulteration, we risk bodily engine failure. For example, many refined foods are designed to give us a quick 'energy fix' by being extra high in calories, but extra low in everything else of nutritional value. To the body, these calories are 'empty calories', using up resources without providing anything of lasting value. If eating empty calories causes us to eat insufficient amounts of other important nutrients, the body simply runs out of resources. What is more, if we eat more energy than we need, then the excess energy may be turned into fat. However, if we eat foods prepared directly by nature, we will eat no empty calories. Natural foods appeal to the senses, with a minimum need for elaborate preparation. They contain such a wealth of vitamins, minerals, fats, oils and proteins that it is nearly impossible to become over- or under-nourished by eating them.

We believe that health is a natural state, and that good food is its basis. To us, people and plants are natural partners on the earth since we use each other's waste products as nourishment. Like the Sioux Indians of old, we recognize that 'all living creatures and all plants derive their life from the sun', because no plant life on earth could exist without the sun and no animal life would survive without plants. We know that a diet based primarily on plants makes it possible for everyone to eat healthily, and that such a diet can be rich, varied and satisfying. If we truly are what we eat, what could be better than eating sunshine?

The experts agree ...

There is so much argument about foods that are bad for us that, on the whole, people do not realize that there is no disagreement about which foods are *good* for us. No nutritional scientist, faced with the body of evidence from around the world, would dispute the fact that a diet based primarily (though not necessarily entirely) on minimally processed and chemically unadulterated fruits, nuts, vegetables, beans and grains is the one most likely to keep a human being healthy in today's world. Taste may dictate an intake of animal derived produce, but that does not alter the basic point: eating more plants makes you healthy:

- There are over 130 pieces of research suggesting that diets high in fruits and vegetables protect against cancer of nearly every susceptible organ in the body.

- Since the early 1960s, research has confirmed that a diet high in natural fibre from vegetables, fruits and unrefined grains protects us from a whole range of 'diseases of civilisation' including diverticulitis, colon cancer, haemorrhoids, gallstones and heart disease.

- Scientists all over the world agree that high intakes of saturated fats from meat and dairy products are linked with coronary heart disease. Expert committees suggest that we should reduce our fat intake and that the simplest way to do this is to eat more plant-based foods.

- There is ample evidence that people following plant-based diets are less likely to suffer from hypertension, late onset diabetes, osteoporosis and kidney stones.

Whose mouth is it anyway?

The World Health Organization has an ambitious definition of health. It is 'the ability of each individual to realize his/her maximum potential for enjoyment of life, with or without infirmity'. Instead of defining health in terms of disease, this is a statement of wellness which stresses the joy of life and emphasizes that health is a personal matter. It accepts that people live in different conditions, with different advantages and difficulties, but it assumes that we *all* have the right to be healthy in our own way.

From the point of view of naturopathic nutrition, no person can give another the gift of health. Physicians and surgeons do wonderful work helping to repair the ravages of modern life, but medicine can only provide good conditions for the body to heal – it cannot actually do the healing. A broken limb can be re-set into the right position, but it is the body that makes the bone ends join together again. Whatever the condition, only nature heals.

By accepting the idea that we are what we eat, we can give our bodies the best possible conditions for health all the time. By saying 'yes' to things that make us healthy more than we say 'yes' to things that do us harm, we can increase our vitality, improve our sense of well-being and reduce the risk of serious illness damaging our lives. Simply by choosing to eat better, we can start to take responsibility for our own health.

CHAPTER THREE

EAT WHAT YOU LIKE

In this chapter, we look at why people choose the foods they eat and discuss the general principles that are the basis of all healthy diets.

For years now, people in the Western world have been eating themselves sick. Up to 400,000 new cancer cases each year are linked with diet, and eighty percent of all cancers may have some relationship to food. High-fat foods increase the risk of coronary heart disease, which causes twenty-seven percent of all deaths in England and Wales. Obesity is associated with high blood pressure, heart attack, diabetes, gallstones, arthritis and chronic chest disease, and diets high in added sugar are a major cause of tooth decay. Research into food and health by leading scientists throughout the world over the past thirty years has proved beyond reasonable doubt that the high-fat, high-sugar, high-protein, high-salt, low-fibre Western diet is bad for individuals and bad for the population as a whole. It is perhaps not surprising, therefore, that there is great interest in the concept of the 'healthy diet', as people prepare to enter the next millennium.

If we ate food simply to satisfy hunger and to nourish our bodies, it would be easy to describe a healthy diet. After all, experts from Europe, North and South America, Australia, New Zealand, Japan and China agree that a healthy diet contains good quantities of fresh fruit and vegetables (including nuts, seeds and pulses) and is relatively low in refined sugars, protein and fat (particularly the saturated fat found in meat and dairy products). A healthy diet provides the energy to do physical and mental work and to resist disease. It appeals to our senses and creates a sense of well-being.

However, the general lack of enthusiasm for actually *eating* a healthy diet in our society suggests that our motives for eating are complicated, and often have nothing to do with health. Here are some of the more common reasons why people eat:

    to express love and caring
    to express individuality
    to demonstrate the nature and extent of our relationships
    to start and maintain business relationships
    to give a focus to group activities
    to show separateness from a group
    to show belonging-ness to a group
    to cope with psychological/emotional stress
    to reward or punish
    to show social status
    to improve self esteem or gain recognition
    to wield political and economic power
    to symbolize powerful emotional experiences
    to display religious feeling
    to represent security
    to express morality
    to signify wealth.   (after Fieldhouse)

These are not the only factors influencing our eating habits. For many people, out-of-date notions about nutrition, combined with the effects of advertising, exert an even greater effect on food choice. For example, before the Second World War, the UK government put considerable effort into persuading people that they should eat less carbohydrate and more protein (including milk, cheese and eggs) to help ensure a so-called balanced diet. Despite the fact that these ideas are now known to be out-of-date and bad for health, people are still influenced by them.

In our view, a diet consisting of healthy food is a healthy diet. To multi-national food companies, however, there is no such thing as good or bad food. They tend to encourage old fashioned ideas about nutrition in an attempt to persuade us that, for example, a profitable protein food, high in salt and fat (like a hot dog) is just as good for us as a protein food low in fat and salt (like soya beans), simply because it *is* a protein food. They suggest that you actually *need* to eat as much meat- and dairy-based foods as you do vegetables, grains and fruits – not because milk and meat foods are particularly good for you, but because they are good for profit.

In most Western countries, the amount of money spent by governments on healthy eating advice and education is less than one fortieth of the money spent on advertising by the food industry, who spend millions each year trying to get us to increase our consumption of their products. As a result, people still believe that balance, variety and moderation in diet are enough to ensure health, even if what is being eaten in a balanced and moderate way is a variety of unhealthy foods.

Realizing that people want to eat for health, but are under pressure to buy unhealthy food, some manufacturers of food supplements suggest that the solution to our dietary health problems is to increase our intake of particular vitamins and minerals. For most people in our society, though, any potential risk of vitamin or mineral deficiency is far outweighed by simple misunderstanding of the basic principles of healthy eating.

As we have said, the basic principles of good nutrition are simple and have stood the test of time; but we also know that the only thing you can change in life is yourself. So rather than suggest just one more 'healthy diet' to be carefully followed and then discarded as impractical after a few months, we want to give you information that you can use to design a healthy diet for yourself. We want you to enjoy eating food that is good for you, rather than painfully cut out foods that are bad for you. We want to help you find healthy foods that you really like, because then the advice we recommend for a healthy diet can be summed up in four words: eat what you like.

We have therefore designed ten Personal Eating Principles which, when applied according to the method described in Part Two, will help you to create a healthy diet that suits your needs, your taste and your pocket. They are based on the wisdom of centuries, but are also in agreement with the most up-to-date recommendations of several international authorities, including the World Health Organization. Over time, eating according to these principles will improve your health and vitality, and give you a new sense of well-being.

Ten personal eating principles

1. Eat enough food to meet your daily energy (calorie) needs.

2. Increase your daily intake of unrefined carbohydrates so that they provide sixty percent or more of your daily energy needs.

3. Adjust your daily intake of fats and oils (most of which should be poly-unsaturated), so that they provide thirty percent or less of your daily energy needs.

4. Adjust your daily intake of protein (whether from plant foods, animal foods, or a combination of the two) to provide about ten percent of your daily energy needs.

5. Increase your daily fibre intake.

6. Reduce your refined sugar, salt and caffeine intakes to the minimum possible level.

7. Try to choose fresh food grown on healthy soil, with a minimum of chemical contamination, and eat your food as close as possible to its original state (raw, wherever possible and palatable).

8. Eat only when you are hungry, chew your food well and don't eat more than you need to feel satisfied.

9. Drink when you are thirsty – and preferably pure water.

10. Allow proper time and space for eating and for enjoying what you eat.

As you will see in Part Two, turning your diet into a healthy way of eating that you really enjoy may take a little time, so here are a few ways that you could start applying the Personal Eating Principles immediately:

- Introduce new, healthy foods into your existing diet (try out some new fruits and vegetables – organic if possible – or eat a little raw salad each day).

- Increase your intake of healthier foods whilst cutting down the intake of some 'unhealthy' foods that are high in fat or sugar (for example, more fruit salad with less cream, more vegetables with less red meat).

- Substitute 'healthy' for 'harmful', (such as some herb tea every now and again in place of tea or coffee, a breakfast cereal with no added sugar instead of an added sugar brand, a low fat product instead of the full fat version).

- Start to choose properly labelled foods, which only contain ingredients that suit your Personal Eating Principles.

- Start writing to food manufacturers asking them to change the ingredients of some of their products to make them better for us.

Change is one of the things that human beings are best at. We change our minds almost every day and so, given proper information, we can change our diet and start eating more healthily. And, however much or little you decide to change your diet, you cannot fail. Any changes you make that are based on the Personal Eating Principles listed above will do you good and will increase your vitality and sense of well-being. What is more, you will be changing in your own way, in your own time and on your own terms.

Eating for health is not a matter of restricting choice. It is a matter of allowing yourself greater personal choice – not to eat what manufacturers tell you to eat, but to eat what *you* have decided is best for you. It is a matter of getting the basics right and making sure that your daily intake of energy, carbohydrate, fat and protein suits your body's needs. If using Personal Eating Principles moves your diet even a little way in the right direction, you will improve your health in the short term and stay healthier in the long term.

Part Two of the book will show you how to make your diet healthier by putting the ten Personal Eating Principles into action.

CHAPTER FOUR

FROM LIGHT TO LIFE

This chapter describes what food is, both chemically and in terms of how it is used by the body. It then looks at the way in which plants manufacture the foods on which we all depend, and at the astonishing variety of foodstuffs that plants provide.

Food basics

The food we eat provides us with the nourishment we need to sustain our lives. Analysed chemically, food consists of a variety of different substances but only some of these – the nutrients – provide us with nutrition. Nutrients provide energy and raw materials for the body and allow our tissues to be built up and broken down according to need.

Nutrients can be divided into five basic categories:

1. Starches and sugars (known as carbohydrates).

2. Fats and oils (sometimes called lipids).

3. Proteins (which are made up of amino acids).

4. Vitamins (such as vitamin C and the B vitamins).

5. Minerals (calcium, magnesium, zinc and so on).

Starches, sugars, fats, oils, proteins, vitamins and edible minerals are made by plants from sunshine, air, earth and water. We can eat them directly as vegetable foods or indirectly as animal foods.

Carbohydrates and fats are mostly used by the body as sources of energy to keep us warm, moving, thinking, digesting and metabolizing.

Proteins are the raw materials – the 'building blocks' – from which body tissues and a huge variety of essential chemicals called enzymes are made. Vegetable foods such as peas, beans, lentils, nuts and cereals contain high levels of protein, as do flesh foods and animal-derived products such as eggs and cheese.

Vitamins are essential chemical co-workers that help the enzymes within body cells control the process of metabolism.

Minerals also play a part in a wide variety of chemical and electrical processes within the body. Both vitamins and minerals are found in many different foodstuffs.

As well as the five basic nutrients, our food contains other non-nutrient substances, such as fibre, water and chemical additives, which can have important effects on health. **Fibre** (nowadays more correctly referred to as non-starch polysaccharide) provides the bulk in food that enables our bowels to work effectively and helps to protect us from bowel disease and high blood cholesterol levels. **Water** from food (together with the water we drink) helps our blood to flow, forms the basis of our body fluids and plays a vital part in our digestion and metabolism. **Chemical additives** affect the appearance, flavour and storage qualities of food and may have an influence on health.

In summary, then, the food we eat contains energy, building blocks, chemical co-workers and non-nutrient substances.

For many people, the art of using good food to provide good nutrition has been over-complicated by too much science. However, the science of digestion and nutrition is really extremely simple. We eat food, break it down in our stomach and intestines, absorb it into our bloodstream and then use it within the body in ways appropriate to our needs at the time. Much of the food we eat is used as fuel for the process of 'internal combustion', which gives us the energy to live, move and stay warm. The rest is used for building or repairing body tissues, and also to provide the chemicals necessary to support our various bodily processes. What we don't use, we eliminate from the body through various channels, usually dissolved in water (as faeces, urine and sweat).

So it is important to remember that being well nourished involves more than just an adequate supply of nutritious food. It also requires healthy digestive organs, a good blood supply and efficient excretory mechanisms for waste products. In other words, whilst there is certainly a difference between healthy food and non-healthy food, there is really no such thing as a 'health food' – that is to say a food that can make you healthy all by itself, just by eating it. Successful nutrition involves paying attention to people as well.

Sunlight and soil

Plants are the basis of all life on earth because they convert light into matter. They form a link between heaven and earth – between sunlight and soil – because they are able to turn the energy of the sun and the earth into forms that we can use to sustain ourselves.

As a plant grows, it uses energy from sunlight, carbon dioxide from the air and water from the environment to produce the carbohydrates which form the basis of the food we eat. This process, which takes place in all green leaves, is known as **photosynthesis** (from the Greek words meaning 'light' and 'to combine into a whole'). Photosynthesis is a miracle of natural recycling.

Carbon dioxide is breathed out into the air as a waste gas by humans and animals. This, plus the carbon dioxide blown into the atmosphere from engines, factories and fires, is taken into the leaves of plants. Here, through the action of sunlight, the carbon is 'reclaimed' from the carbon dioxide and made into carbohydrate by photosynthesis. As part of the process, oxygen is produced as a 'waste product' and this re-stocks the atmosphere with the oxygen we need to breathe. Plants and animals therefore live in a perfectly balanced relationship, because they recycle each other's waste products.

Since all living things on earth are built on carbon, and since most of the energy used by human beings is produced by burning carbon in one form or another, it is no exaggeration to say that, without green plants 'fixing' carbon from the air by photosynthesis, there would be no life.

To help achieve photosynthesis, plants suck up water (together with fertilizer and minerals) from the earth by creating an unbroken column of liquid all the way up through the roots, stems and branches and up to the leaves. This water is not used up, but is evaporated from the leaves into the air, eventually to become clouds and fall as rain, ready to be used again.

Plants make sunlight available for us to use as energy, and in the process produce a myriad of other materials necessary for healthy life. Just as remarkable, they enable us to share in the goodness of the soil by turning the raw materials of earth into edible nutrients, such as proteins, oils and minerals, which we can use to build and repair our bodies. Plants are our link to the vital energies of the sun and the earth.

Green foodstores

Naturopathic nutrition is about following nature's laws and, when it comes to eating, the best way for us to do this is to base our diet on the huge variety of plant foods that nature provides. You only have to think of the strength and beauty of a horse in peak condition or the magnificent physique of a mountain gorilla to understand the health giving potential of a plant-based diet. Nature's example is to eat plenty of varied, unadulterated, locally grown fresh foods in season, with a minimum of preparation.

Plant foods as a group contain all the nutrients necessary for human health and vitality. They are naturally high in the right sorts of fibre and low in cholesterol. Plant foods are our only source of energy-giving complex carbohydrates and contain no refined sugar. They contain no saturated or trans fats (see page 193), and are naturally high in health-giving polyunsaturates. Plant foods contain all essential amino acids and essential fatty acids. They help to protect against all major cancers (except, perhaps, prostate cancer) and against diseases of the heart and digestive system. Plant foods are tasty, inexpensive and can be enjoyed with minimum preparation. They take relatively little room to grow. They are available to us in huge variety and the different parts of plants provide us with an astonishing variety of foodstuffs.

Roots anchor plants in the ground and gather up water, fertilizer and minerals from the soil. They act as storage space for energy during winter months and provide foods such as carrots, beetroots, parsnips and other biennial root vegetables.

Stems provide a roadway between the top and bottom of plants and are also used to store energy. Celery and fennel are both edible examples of stem foods.

Leaves are the production power-houses of plants, where carbohydrates, proteins, oils and vitamins are made. Green leaves such as spinach, parsley and salads are therefore amongst the most vital foods we can eat.

Flowers provide the means by which the next generation of plants is produced, and many contain important vitamins and oils. Broccoli, cauliflower and artichoke are examples of flower foods.

Fruits and Berries are made by plants to conceal seeds, in the hope of attracting animals to eat the fruits and deposit the seeds elsewhere, thereby helping the species to spread and survive. Fruits and berries contain a wealth of vitamins and minerals and provide a dazzling variety of flavours and textures – such as peaches, oranges, strawberries, blackberries, pineapples, bananas, apples, dates, figs, passion fruits, as well as olives, avocados, peppers, courgettes, aubergines, cucumbers, pumpkins and tomatoes.

Nuts are seeds covered with a hard shell instead of with a soft fruit, and provide another way of making sure that plant seeds are distributed as widely as possible. Nuts such as brazil nuts, cashews, hazelnuts, almonds and walnuts contain important oils as well as vitamins and minerals, and are concentrated sources of protein.

Seeds which are dropped to the ground or onto the wind by plants provide a huge variety of foods, rich in energy, protein, oils, vitamins and minerals. They include grains such as wheat, oats, barley and rye; beans, pulses and peas; sunflower and sesame seeds, to name but a few.

It is clear that a diet based on plant foods can be varied, tasty, nutritious and good for our health. The question is, how much do we need to eat of which foods to be absolutely sure of getting all the nourishment we need?

CHAPTER FIVE

HOW MUCH IS ENOUGH?

This chapter describes the concept of 'Dietary Reference Values' and discusses ways of ensuring that we obtain all the necessary nutrients from our diet.

Ever since the Second World War, panels of experts have wrestled with the problem of defining how much we need of various nutrients to remain healthy. In 1969, the UK Department of Health and Social Security produced *Recommended Intakes for Nutrients*, followed in 1979 by the publication of *Recommended Daily Amounts* (RDAs). However, despite the efforts of the scientists who compiled them, the meaning of these figures was misunderstood by the wider public. Instead of seeing them as crude tools for assessing the general adequacy of the diet of the population *as a whole*, people took them to represent recommendations for intakes of different nutrients suitable for *individuals*. RDAs were deliberately set high, on the grounds that this would help to minimize the risk of any nutrient deficiencies occurring in the population. The experts tried to explain that almost nobody needed to eat the full RDA of all nutrients to be healthy, but unfortunately their words were largely ignored. People came to believe that if they were consuming less than the RDA of a particular nutrient, then they were deficient in that nutrient.

This is not true. RDAs are not a standard against which to assess an individual diet – they are guidelines which help scientists to assess the general nutritional status of large groups of people.

In fact, the question 'How much of this nutrient do I need to be healthy?' is, in scientific terms, extraordinarily difficult to answer. Firstly, medical science has no generally agreed definition of health. Secondly, people vary enormously in their individual needs for particular nutrients, because their bodies, lives and circumstances are so very different. Thirdly, the proportion of a nutrient that is actually absorbed from food by the body varies greatly from person to person and from nutrient to nutrient. Fourthly, the risks and benefits of eating more than the amount necessary to avoid a deficiency of a particular nutrient are not well understood. In the end, whatever figures you choose, some people are going to need more and others less.

Recognizing this unsatisfactory state of affairs, the UK Chief Medical Officer asked the *Committee on Medical Aspects of Food Policy* (COMA) to look into the issue of dietary reference standards. COMA appointed a group of experts to review all the available evidence on human nutritional needs and, in 1991, they published a new set of figures called Dietary Reference Values (DRVs). Unlike RDAs, which are single recommended amounts for daily nutrient intakes, Dietary Reference Values (DRVs) consist of several different figures for each nutrient. These are:

1. Estimated Average Requirements (EARs) – an estimate of the average requirement of an average healthy person.

2. Reference Nutrient Intakes (RNIs) – amounts of each nutrient so high that nobody eating them could become deficient. RNIs are much higher than most people actually need, and are at the top end of a range of values.

3. Lower Reference Nutrient Intakes (LRNIs) – amounts of each nutrient so low that anybody eating less is likely to be deficient; in other words, the bottom end of a range of values.

4. Safe Intakes – amounts of particular nutrients considered to be adequate for most people's needs, but not high enough to be dangerous. Safe intakes are quoted when there is not enough information available to estimate EARs, RNIs and LRNIs.

By using the term 'reference intakes' instead of 'recommended intakes', the UK experts hoped that people would use their figures as general points of reference instead of as definitive values. They also hoped that Dietary Reference Values would be used to help in the assessment of the diet of groups of people, in the development of national food policies, and to make nutrition information on food labels more meaningful.

By providing LRNIs, they tried to give figures of relevance to individual diets, as someone eating less than the LRNI of a particular nutrient is indeed likely to have a deficiency in it. By recommending the use of the term 'non-starch polysaccharide' instead of the old fashioned 'dietary fibre', they also emphasized that the 'non-digestible' parts of plant foods have a variety of important effects on individual health (see pages 67 to 70).

However, although UK Dietary Reference Values try to take account of the fact that people have very different nutritional requirements, like the RDAs they were intended to replace, DRVs are still primarily a guide to population nutrition, not individual nutrition. They also suffer from the fact that, with up to three different standards being given for each nutrient, people still tend to fix on just one figure as the 'recommended' amount.

The result is that, despite all the hard work and clear thinking of the experts, much of the old confusion about nutrient intakes persists in the minds of consumers and food producers. This must be a great frustration to the COMA panel, who gave the following clear warning:

'... for *most* nutrients, there were *insufficient data to set the EAR or LRNI or RNI or safe intake with any great confidence.* Some of the data used in deriving the figures are based on dietary surveys which, in themselves, are not absolutely precise' (our italics)

So, according to expert scientists, Dietary Reference Values are mostly guesstimates and assumptions which cannot be relied on as a guide for individual nutritional needs.

The problem of defining useful Dietary Reference Values is not confined to the UK and nutritional scientists in the United States, the European Union, Australia, New Zealand and South Africa have all faced similar difficulties. The World Health Organization recognizes that DRVs applicable to affluent Westerners may be quite inappropriate to the circumstances of many people in the non-industrialized South and, as a result, they have tried to develop dietary guidelines that take a world perspective.

Even when it *is* possible to make precise theoretical recommendations of nutrient intakes, it is hard to convert these recommendations into practical dietary advice. This is because different foods – processed and prepared in so many different ways – vary so much in their nutritional composition. Also, when practical dietary advice is given, there is always the risk that people will take no notice if the advice demands a bigger dietary change than they are prepared to make (for reasons of taste, convenience or price).

How, then, is it possible to work out how much to eat of which foods, if we want to be healthy? From the point of view of naturopathic nutrition, the first step is to realize that, in our society, we are not suffering from a deficiency of individual nutrients; we are suffering from a deficiency of good nutrition! Except in very unusual circumstances, the chances of anybody who is eating a Western diet developing a *particular* nutrient deficiency are very small. Yet the chances of suffering the ill effects of dietary excess – obesity, coronary heart disease, strokes, cancer and bowel disorders – are extremely high. All these conditions are related to a deficiency of good diet, not a deficiency of individual nutrients. They are associated with eating too much saturated fat, too much sugar and, in some cases, too much protein. These conditions are certainly not related to a lack of nutritional supplements. So, whatever country we live in, instead of worrying about how *much* we are eating of particular nutrients compared with the 'recommended' amounts, we should start concentrating on *what* we are eating.

The next step is to realize that plants provide nutrients in extraordinarily well-balanced packages. That this is not more widely understood is partly a result of the way that nutrition tables are written. When the nutrient content of a food is expressed in terms of grams of nutrient per hundred grams of food, plant foods may appear not to offer as much nutritional value as non-plant foods. However, what matters in nutritional terms is what percentage of the energy (calories) of the food is provided by the nutrient in question. For example, if ten percent of your total calorie intake comes from protein, you will be eating more than enough protein to maintain your health. So, if the foods you eat contain, on average, about ten percent of their calories in the form of protein, you will always eat enough protein as long as you eat enough food to cover your energy needs (in other words, enough to satisfy your hunger).

One hundred grams of potatoes contains, on average, 1.8 grams of protein, which may not seem much. However, ten percent of the calories of a potato come from its protein content. Fresh peas and beans contain about 3.9 grams of protein per 100 grams, but thirty-seven percent of the calories in peas and beans come from their protein content. Even the humble lettuce contains twenty-three percent of its calories in the form of protein.

Therefore, although the nutrients in plant foods may not be highly concentrated (because plants contain a lot of water), plants are extremely rich in essential nutrients and can easily provide for all your nutritional needs *as long as you eat enough of them to give you all the calories you need.* As we have said, horses could not build their beautiful muscular bodies if they weren't getting enough protein, and they only eat grasses. The point is, they eat a *lot* of grasses. Enough grasses to meet their daily calorie requirements.

Naturopathic nutrition is about improving the quality of what you are eating and thereby improving the quality of your life and health. Its method is simple, cheap and available to everyone. Instead of asking you to perform complex calculations, naturopathic nutrition simply recommends that you eat a certain number of portions of your choice of a wide variety of healthy foods each week. If you do this, you will unavoidably eat all you need of all essential nutrients, and naturally tend to avoid things that do you harm. It's as easy as that.

The next two chapters will take you step-by-step through the process of recording and analysing your own diet and describe how to start applying the Personal Eating Principles given in Chapter Three. All you will need is a pen or pencil and some sheets of paper, and a determination to start eating for health.

CHAPTER SIX

KEEPING A DIET DIARY

In this chapter, we describe – with examples – how to draw up and analyse a seven-day diet diary, and give a simple way of summarizing your weekly food intake.

One of the unique features of naturopathic nutrition is that it classifies foods into natural groups, based on how they grow. It recognizes that all foods taken from the same parts of plants – tubers, bulbs, roots stems, leaves, flowers, seeds, fruits or berries – have similar nutritional contents, and this basic observation makes it possible to simplify the process of diet analysis.

Instead of wading through page after page of complicated food composition tables, the naturopathic nutrition method of diet analysis makes it easy to assess the nutritional quality of any individual diet simply by seeing how much food from each natural food group has been eaten during a week. Grouping foods in a natural way also allows greater personal choice when it comes to improving diet, which simply involves adjusting the proportions of foods eaten from each food group.

However, since a journey of a thousand miles starts with the ground under your feet, the first step to improving your diet is to build up an accurate picture of your current eating habits; and the easiest way to do this is to keep a seven-day diet diary.

A seven-day diet diary

Keeping a seven-day diet diary involves writing down everything you eat or drink, as soon as you have eaten or drunk it, every day for seven days.

Take seven pieces of A5 paper (loose-leaf or in a notebook, as convenient). Mark the first piece Monday, the next Tuesday and so on until you have one piece for each of the seven days.

Then draw a line half-way down each sheet and another line that divides the bottom half in half again. Head the top space 'Food and Drink', the second space 'Alcohol and Smoking' and the third space 'Exercise'. Like this:

<table>
<tr><td>

MONDAY
Food and Drink

</td></tr>
<tr><td>

Alcohol and Smoking

</td></tr>
<tr><td>

Exercise

</td></tr>
</table>

Each day for seven consecutive days, carry the appropriate piece of paper and a pencil with you everywhere you go. Every time you eat something, or have a non-alcoholic drink, write it down under Food and Drink. You don't have to weigh or measure anything – just record every *helping* of every food or drink you consume.

For bread, biscuits and cakes, give the number of pieces you ate. With yoghurts or other things in individual serving packs, give the number of pots or packets. For dishes that contain a mixture of ingredients, record each ingredient as a separate helping eg. spaghetti with tomato and mushroom sauce would be written: 1 spaghetti, 1 tomatoes, 1 onions, 1 mushrooms, 1 oil, 1 garlic and 1 herbs. Don't worry if you don't know all the ingredients – just record those that you do know, or that are obvious from looking at the dish. And don't wait until the end of the day to fill up the sheet. Do it straight after every meal or snack.

If you drink any alcohol or smoke any cigarettes, cigars or pipes that day, record these under 'Alcohol' and 'Smoking'.

If you take any exercise – lasting five minutes or more – write it down under the 'Exercise' heading, together with a note of how long the exercise lasted. (Walking, gardening, DIY and sex all count as exercise as long as they make you a bit breathless or sweaty.)

An example of a completed record sheet for one day is given on the next page. Remember, the numbers refer to how many helpings, slices, servings, packets or pots were eaten of the food in question. 1 grapes means one helping of grapes, not one grape.

When each day's sheet is complete, store it safely away until you have collected all seven. And remember, you have nothing to lose by being absolutely honest. No-one is going to read the sheets except you and, in the end, it is still going to be entirely up to you what you eat and how much you eat.

The seven-day diet diary – questions and answers

Q. *Wouldn't it be much easier and quicker to just sit down and try and remember everything I ate during the past seven days?*

A. No. Very few people can remember their food intake in detail beyond a couple of days ago. What's more, although most of us think that we already know what we eat each week, what we believe we eat and what we really eat are often surprisingly different from each other.

Q. *Seven days seems rather a long time to be scribbling things on bits of paper after each meal or snack; wouldn't two or three days be enough?*

A. If you want to make a meaningful assessment of the nutritional value of your diet, you have to take account of two things. First, being creatures of variety, we tend to eat different things on different days according to our changing circumstances. Second, as creatures of habit with particular likes and dislikes, our diets have repeating patterns in them. A seven-day diet diary usually makes these patterns clear and gives a reasonably accurate impression of the full range of foods we consume.

Q. *I'd like to start today, but this week is going to be a bit unusual. Shouldn't I wait for a normal week before doing my seven-day diet diary?*

MONDAY
Food and Drink

I Allbran
I Yoghurt
I Grapes
2 Ryvitas
2 Marmite
2 Butter
2 Cups herb tea
I Green salad
I Cup of black coffee
I Cheese
I Vinaigrette dressing
I Satsuma
2 Digestive biscuits
I Cup of tea
I Baked trout
I Potatoes
I Courgettes

Exercise

¾ Hour swimming
Sex

Alcohol and Smoking

2 Brandy and sodas

A. People's average food intake stays more or less the same whether their week is 'normal' or 'abnormal'. Nearly every week has some reason for not being normal, and waiting for a normal week before starting a seven-day diet diary might mean never starting at all. Our advice is, if you want to assess your diet, do it straightaway.

Q. *Why do I have to record my alcohol intake, smoking and exercise?*

A. It is entirely up to you how much alcohol you drink, how much you smoke and how much exercise you take. The reason we suggest making a separate note of your tobacco, alcohol and exercise habits is so that you can take stock and decide for yourself whether they should be modified.

If your objective is optimum health, there is absolutely no question that you should not smoke and that you should take moderate, regular exercise (suitable to your age and general level of fitness). Similarly, alcohol is a proven risk to health in all but the most moderate amounts and, glass for glass, is a potent way of consuming more calories than you need at the expense of good nutrition.

We know that changing these habits requires great determination and will-power though, especially in the early stages. Luckily, a general improvement in diet and nutrition in itself seems to reduce the attractions of alcohol and tobacco for many people, and the extra sense of vitality gained from eating well is often enough to encourage the taking of some more exercise.

Analysing your seven-day diet diary

Once you have collected your seven record sheets, here is a simple way to analyse them and to condense all the information about your present eating habits into one simple chart.

Starting on page 32 of this chapter, you will find a specially designed Diet Analysis Chart. This consists of a list of different foods and drinks – divided into groups – with a row of numbers under each group, eg:

1. Roots and Tubers
1a. Beetroot, carrot, celeriac, parsnip, swede, turnip
    1 2 3 4 5 6 7 8 9 10 11 12 13 14 15 16 17 18 19 20 21 22 23 24 25

Take a few moments now to study this chart.

Next, take the first page of your diet diary and find the first thing that you ate that day. Look for the food group containing this particular food in the Diet Analysis Chart and then cross out the number of helpings you ate of this food. For example, if your first recorded food was two slices of white toast, you would mark the chart like this:

iii) Breads (brown, white, wholemeal, rye)
     1̸ 2̸ 3 4 5 6 7 8 9 10 11 12 13 14 15 16 17 18 19 20 21 22 23 24 25
     26 27 28 29 30 31 32 33 34 35 36 37 38 39 40 41 42 43 44 45 46 47 48

If the next thing you ate was 1 bowl of porridge, you would cross out the number 1 under group 6b.v), Sugar-free breakfast cereals. If you had some milk with your porridge, you would also cross out the number 1 under group 12a, Milk and milk products.

Carry on like this through the rest of your diet diary, crossing out numbers under the appropriate food groups for every helping of food you ate (and also for every cup or glass of drink you had). If you ate a food that is not on the list, mark it off under the category that you feel comes closest. Using this method, it is easy to see exactly what you ate and drank during the week in question, because the last number crossed out on any particular line in the chart gives you the total number of helpings you ate or drank from that group during the week.

DIET ANALYSIS CHART

1. Roots and Tubers
1a. Beetroot, carrot, celeriac, parsnip, swede, turnip
     1 2 3 4 5 6 7 8 9 10 11 12 13 14 15 16 17 18 19 20 21 22 23 24 25
1b. All potatoes, sweet potatoes, yams
     1 2 3 4 5 6 7 8 9 10 11 12 13 14 15 16 17 18 19 20 21 22 23 24 25
1c. Ginger
     1 2 3 4 5 6 7 8 9 10 11 12 13 14 15 16 17 18 19 20 21 22 23 24 25
1d. Horseradish
     1 2 3 4 5 6 7 8 9 10 11 12 13 14 15 16 17 18 19 20 21 22 23 24 25
1e. Radishes
     1 2 3 4 5 6 7 8 9 10 11 12 13 14 15 16 17 18 19 20 21 22 23 24 25
2. Bulbs
2a. Onions, shallots, spring onions, leeks
     1 2 3 4 5 6 7 8 9 10 11 12 13 14 15 16 17 18 19 20 21 22 23 24 25
2b. Garlic
     1 2 3 4 5 6 7 8 9 10 11 12 13 14 15 16 17 18 19 20 21 22 23 24 25
3. Stems
3a. Celery, fennel
     1 2 3 4 5 6 7 8 9 10 11 12 13 14 15 16 17 18 19 20 21 22 23 24 25

DIET ANALYSIS CHART, *continued*

4. Leaves

4a. Greens (brussels sprouts, cabbage, curly kale, endive, spinach, spring greens)

    1 2 3 4 5 6 7 8 9 10 11 12 13 14 15 16 17 18 19 20 21 22 23 24 25

4b. Salads (all lettuces)

    1 2 3 4 5 6 7 8 9 10 11 12 13 14 15 16 17 18 19 20 21 22 23 24 25

4c. Cress (mustard and cress, watercress)

    1 2 3 4 5 6 7 8 9 10 11 12 13 14 15 16 17 18 19 20 21 22 23 24 25

4d. Herbs (basil, chives, coriander, dill, mint, oregano, parsley, rosemary, sage, tarragon, thyme)

    1 2 3 4 5 6 7 8 9 10 11 12 13 14 15 16 17 18 19 20 21 22 23 24 25

5. Flowers

5a. Artichoke, asparagus, cauliflower, green broccoli, purple broccoli

    1 2 3 4 5 6 7 8 9 10 11 12 13 14 15 16 17 18 19 20 21 22 23 24 25

6. Seeds

6a. Pulses

  i) Fresh Pulses (broad beans, green beans, runner beans, mange tout, all peas)

    1 2 3 4 5 6 7 8 9 10 11 12 13 14 15 16 17 18 19 20 21 22 23 24 25

  ii) Sprouts

    1 2 3 4 5 6 7 8 9 10 11 12 13 14 15 16 17 18 19 20 21 22 23 24 25

  iii) Dried Pulses (aduki beans, black gram, blackeye beans, butter beans, chick-peas, etc.)

    1 2 3 4 5 6 7 8 9 10 11 12 13 14 15 16 17 18 19 20 21 22 23 24 25

  iv) Lentils (red, green, brown, dal, etc.)

    1 2 3 4 5 6 7 8 9 10 11 12 13 14 15 16 17 18 19 20 21 22 23 24 25

  v) Soya products (soya beans, tempeh, tofu)

    1 2 3 4 5 6 7 8 9 10 11 12 13 14 15 16 17 18 19 20 21 22 23 24 25

  vi) Soya milk

    1 2 3 4 5 6 7 8 9 10 11 12 13 14 15 16 17 18 19 20 21 22 23 24 25

  vii) Baked beans

    1 2 3 4 5 6 7 8 9 10 11 12 13 14 15 16 17 18 19 20 21 22 23 24 25

  viii) Hummus

    1 2 3 4 5 6 7 8 9 10 11 12 13 14 15 16 17 18 19 20 21 22 23 24 25

6b. Grains

  i) Wholegrains and flours (barley, buckwheat, bulgur, couscous, millet, rye, wheat)

    1 2 3 4 5 6 7 8 9 10 11 12 13 14 15 16 17 18 19 20 21 22 23 24 25

  ii) Rice products (brown rice, white rice, basmati, rice flour)

    1 2 3 4 5 6 7 8 9 10 11 12 13 14 15 16 17 18 19 20 21 22 23 24 25

DIET ANALYSIS CHART, *continued*

6b. Grains, cont.

  iii) Breads (brown, white, wholemeal, rye)

    1 2 3 4 5 6 7 8 9 10 11 12 13 14 15 16 17 18 19 20 21 22 23 24 25
    26 27 28 29 30 31 32 33 34 35 36 37 38 39 40 41 42 43 44 45 46 47 48

  iv) Pasta (macaroni, spaghetti, tagliatelle, etc.)

    1 2 3 4 5 6 7 8 9 10 11 12 13 14 15 16 17 18 19 20 21 22 23 24 25

  v) Sugar-free breakfast cereals (sugar-free muesli, porridge)

    1 2 3 4 5 6 7 8 9 10 11 12 13 14 15 16 17 18 19 20 21 22 23 24 25

  vi) Other breakfast cereals

    1 2 3 4 5 6 7 8 9 10 11 12 13 14 15 16 17 18 19 20 21 22 23 24 25

  vii) Miscellaneous grain products (bran, cornflour, oatmeal, oatcakes, sago, semolina, sweetcorn, wheatgerm, etc.)

    1 2 3 4 5 6 7 8 9 10 11 12 13 14 15 16 17 18 19 20 21 22 23 24 25

6c. Spices

  i) Anise, caraway, celery seed, coriander, cumin, dill, fennel, mustard, etc.

    1 2 3 4 5 6 7 8 9 10 11 12 13 14 15 16 17 18 19 20 21 22 23 24 25

6d. Nuts and seeds

  i) Almonds, brazils, cashews, hazels, peanuts, pecans, pine kernels, pumpkin seeds, sesame seeds, sunflower seeds, walnuts (including nut butters)

    1 2 3 4 5 6 7 8 9 10 11 12 13 14 15 16 17 18 19 20 21 22 23 24 25

  ii) Coconut

    1 2 3 4 5 6 7 8 9 10 11 12 13 14 15 16 17 18 19 20 21 22 23 24 25

7. Fruits

7a. Vegetable fruits

  i) Aubergine, courgette, cucumber, marrow, pepper, pumpkin, squash, tomato

    1 2 3 4 5 6 7 8 9 10 11 12 13 14 15 16 17 18 19 20 21 22 23 24 25

  ii) Avocado

    1 2 3 4 5 6 7 8 9 10 11 12 13 14 15 16 17 18 19 20 21 22 23 24 25

  iii) Okra

    1 2 3 4 5 6 7 8 9 10 11 12 13 14 15 16 17 18 19 20 21 22 23 24 25

  iv) Olives

    1 2 3 4 5 6 7 8 9 10 11 12 13 14 15 16 17 18 19 20 21 22 23 24 25

7b. Sweet fruits

  i) Apples and pears (all types)

    1 2 3 4 5 6 7 8 9 10 11 12 13 14 15 16 17 18 19 20 21 22 23 24 25

  ii) Melons (all types)

    1 2 3 4 5 6 7 8 9 10 11 12 13 14 15 16 17 18 19 20 21 22 23 24 25

  iii) Tropical fruits (mango, pawpaw, banana, passion, pineapple)

    1 2 3 4 5 6 7 8 9 10 11 12 13 14 15 16 17 18 19 20 21 22 23 24 25

DIET ANALYSIS CHART, *continued*

7b. Sweet fruits, cont.

  iv) Soft fruits (apricots, peaches, plums, nectarines, sharon fruit, grapes, cherries)

    1 2 3 4 5 6 7 8 9 10 11 12 13 14 15 16 17 18 19 20 21 22 23 24 25

7c. Citrus fruits (clementine, grapefruit, lemon, orange, satsuma, tangerine)

    1 2 3 4 5 6 7 8 9 10 11 12 13 14 15 16 17 18 19 20 21 22 23 24 25

7d. Dried fruits (apricots, dates, figs, prunes, raisins, sultanas, etc.)

    1 2 3 4 5 6 7 8 9 10 11 12 13 14 15 16 17 18 19 20 21 22 23 24 25

8. Berries

8a. Blackberries, blackcurrants, cranberries, gooseberries, raspberries, redcurrants, strawberries

    1 2 3 4 5 6 7 8 9 10 11 12 13 14 15 16 17 18 19 20 21 22 23 24 25

9. Fungi

9a. All types of mushroom

    1 2 3 4 5 6 7 8 9 10 11 12 13 14 15 16 17 18 19 20 21 22 23 24 25

10. Oils

10a. Oils high in saturates (coconut, palm, animal fats and oils)

    1 2 3 4 5 6 7 8 9 10 11 12 13 14 15 16 17 18 19 20 21 22 23 24 25

10b. Oils high in mono-unsaturates (hazelnut, olive, peanut)

    1 2 3 4 5 6 7 8 9 10 11 12 13 14 15 16 17 18 19 20 21 22 23 24 25

10c. Oils high in polyunsaturates (corn, evening primrose, grapeseed, safflower, sesame, soya, sunflower, vegetable, walnut, wheatgerm)

    1 2 3 4 5 6 7 8 9 10 11 12 13 14 15 16 17 18 19 20 21 22 23 24 25

10d. Polyunsaturated margarines (containing no hydrogenated fats)

    1 2 3 4 5 6 7 8 9 10 11 12 13 14 15 16 17 18 19 20 21 22 23 24 25

10e. Other margarines

    1 2 3 4 5 6 7 8 9 10 11 12 13 14 15 16 17 18 19 20 21 22 23 24 25

11. Miscellaneous Plant Products

11a. Yeast extracts (eg. Marmite)

    1 2 3 4 5 6 7 8 9 10 11 12 13 14 15 16 17 18 19 20 21 22 23 24 25

11b. Soya sauce

    1 2 3 4 5 6 7 8 9 10 11 12 13 14 15 16 17 18 19 20 21 22 23 24 25

11c. Vinegar

    1 2 3 4 5 6 7 8 9 10 11 12 13 14 15 16 17 18 19 20 21 22 23 24 25

11d. Seaweeds

    1 2 3 4 5 6 7 8 9 10 11 12 13 14 15 16 17 18 19 20 21 22 23 24 25

12. Dairy

12a. Milk and milk products (all types of cow, goat and sheep milk, cheese and yoghurt)

    1 2 3 4 5 6 7 8 9 10 11 12 13 14 15 16 17 18 19 20 21 22 23 24 25

12b. Eggs (all types)

    1 2 3 4 5 6 7 8 9 10 11 12 13 14 15 16 17 18 19 20 21 22 23 24 25

DIET ANALYSIS CHART, *continued*

13. Meats

13a. Meat (beef, lamb, pork, venison, etc.)

1 2 3 4 5 6 7 8 9 10 11 12 13 14 15 16 17 18 19 20 21 22 23 24 25

13b. Fowl (chicken, duck, game birds, goose, turkey)

1 2 3 4 5 6 7 8 9 10 11 12 13 14 15 16 17 18 19 20 21 22 23 24 25

13c. Processed meat and offal (all dried, cured and processed meats – ham, salami, sausages, meat pies, etc. – plus all offal products, ie. brawn, heart, liver, kidney, etc.)

1 2 3 4 5 6 7 8 9 10 11 12 13 14 15 16 17 18 19 20 21 22 23 24 25

14. Fish

14a. Lean fish (cod, plaice, whiting, sole, etc.)

1 2 3 4 5 6 7 8 9 10 11 12 13 14 15 16 17 18 19 20 21 22 23 24 25

14b. Oily fish (herring, mackerel, salmon, etc.)

1 2 3 4 5 6 7 8 9 10 11 12 13 14 15 16 17 18 19 20 21 22 23 24 25

14c. Shellfish (all types)

1 2 3 4 5 6 7 8 9 10 11 12 13 14 15 16 17 18 19 20 21 22 23 24 25

15. Drinks

15a. Water

1 2 3 4 5 6 7 8 9 10 11 12 13 14 15 16 17 18 19 20 21 22 23 24 25

15b. Pure fruit juice

1 2 3 4 5 6 7 8 9 10 11 12 13 14 15 16 17 18 19 20 21 22 23 24 25

15c. Soft drinks and mixers

1 2 3 4 5 6 7 8 9 10 11 12 13 14 15 16 17 18 19 20 21 22 23 24 25

15d. Caffeinated beverages (tea, coffee, etc.)

1 2 3 4 5 6 7 8 9 10 11 12 13 14 15 16 17 18 19 20 21 22 23 24 25

15e. Caffeine-free beverages (herb teas, dandelion 'coffees', roast barley 'coffees', etc.)

1 2 3 4 5 6 7 8 9 10 11 12 13 14 15 16 17 18 19 20 21 22 23 24 25

16. Sweet Foods and Snacks

16a. All types of confectionery (sweets, chocolates, candies, etc.)

1 2 3 4 5 6 7 8 9 10 11 12 13 14 15 16 17 18 19 20 21 22 23 24 25

16b. Sugar, syrups and spreads (sugar, cane syrup, maple syrup, jam, marmalade, honey)

1 2 3 4 5 6 7 8 9 10 11 12 13 14 15 16 17 18 19 20 21 22 23 24 25

16c. Cakes and biscuits (all types)

1 2 3 4 5 6 7 8 9 10 11 12 13 14 15 16 17 18 19 20 21 22 23 24 25

16d. Savoury snacks (crisps, etc.)

1 2 3 4 5 6 7 8 9 10 11 12 13 14 15 16 17 18 19 20 21 22 23 24 25

Recording Your Portion Totals

Now you have filled in your Diet Analysis Chart, use it to fill in the blanks in the following Portion Totals Chart. You will need this information in the next chapter to assess the nutritional quality of your diet.

PORTION TOTALS CHART

Food Group	Your Weekly Portion Total
1. Roots and Tubers	
1a. Beetroot, carrot, etc.	_____
1b. Potatoes, etc.	_____
1c. Ginger	_____
1d. Horseradish	_____
1e. Radishes	_____
2. Bulbs	
2a. Onions, etc.	_____
2b. Garlic	_____
3. Stems	
3a. Celery, fennel	_____
4. Leaves	
4a. Greens (brussels sprouts, curly kale, etc.)	_____
4b. Salads (all lettuces)	_____
4c. Cress (mustard and cress, watercress)	_____
4d. Herbs (basil, chives, dill, etc.)	_____
5. Flowers	
5a. Artichokes, etc.	_____
6. Seeds	
6a. Pulses	
i) Fresh Pulses (green beans, peas, etc.)	_____
ii) Sprouts	_____
iii) Dried Pulses (beans, chick-peas, split peas, etc.)	_____

PORTION TOTALS CHART, *continued*

Food Group	Your Weekly Portion Total
6a. Pulses, cont.	
iv) Lentils	_____
v) Soya products	_____
vi) Soya milk	_____
vii) Baked beans	_____
viii) Hummus	_____
6b. Grains	
i) Wholegrains and flours (wheat, barley, etc.)	_____
ii) Rice products (brown, white, basmati)	_____
iii) Breads (brown, white, wholemeal, rye)	_____
iv) Pasta (spaghetti, macaroni, tagliatelle, etc.)	_____
v) Sugar-free breakfast cereals	_____
vi) Other breakfast cereals	_____
vii) Miscellaneous grain products	_____
6c. Spices (anise, caraway, etc.)	_____
6d. Nuts and seeds	
i) Almonds, brazils, etc.	_____
ii) Coconut	_____

7. Fruits

7a. Vegetable fruits	
i) Aubergine, courgette, etc.	_____
ii) Avocado	_____
iii) Okra	_____
iv) Olives	_____
7b. Sweet Fruits	
i) Apples and pears (all types)	_____
ii) Melons (all types)	_____
iii) Tropical fruits (mango, banana, etc.)	_____
iv) Soft fruits (apricots, peaches, plums, etc.)	_____

PORTION TOTALS CHART, *continued*

Food Group	Your Weekly Portion Total
7c. Citrus fruits (all types)	_____
7d. Dried fruits (apricots, dates, etc.)	_____

8. Berries

8a. Blackberries, blackcurrants, etc.	_____

9. Fungi

9a. All types of mushroom	_____

10. Oils

10a. Oils high in saturates	_____
10b. Oils high in mono-unsaturates	_____
10c. Oils high in polyunsaturates	_____
10d. Polyunsaturated margarines	_____
10e. Other margarines	_____

11. Miscellaneous Plant Products

11a. Yeast extract (eg. Marmite)	_____
11b. Soya sauce	_____
11c. Vinegar	_____
11d. Seaweeds	_____

12. Dairy

12a. Milk and milk products	_____
12b. Eggs (all types)	_____

13. Meats

13a. Meat	_____
13b. Fowl	_____
13c. Processed meat and offal	_____

14. Fish

14a. Lean fish	_____
14b. Oily fish	_____
14c. Shellfish	_____

PORTION TOTALS CHART, *continued*

Food Group   *Your Weekly Portion Total*

15. Drinks

15a. Water   _____

15b. Pure fruit juice   _____

15c. Soft drinks and mixers   _____

15d. Caffeinated beverages   _____

15e. Caffeine-free beverages   _____

16. Sweet Foods and Snacks

16a. Confectionary   _____

16b. Sugar, syrups and spreads   _____

16c. Cakes and biscuits   _____

16d. Savoury snacks   _____

Now that you have completed and analysed your seven-day diet diary and filled in the weekly Portion Totals Charts above, you are in a position to use the method described in the following chapter to assess the nutritional value of your present diet. You can then start applying the ten Personal Eating Principles mentioned in Part One to create a new, healthier diet for yourself, a diet which will increase your vitality and give you a new sense of well-being.

CHAPTER SEVEN

PRACTICAL NATUROPATHIC NUTRITION

In this chapter, we explain how to apply the ten Personal Eating Principles given in Chapter Three.

At the end of Part One, we listed ten Personal Eating Principles designed to help you improve your health and vitality simply by eating better (see pages 14–15). There is widespread agreement amongst nutritionists and other health care professionals that eating according to such principles is good for health and likely to reduce the risk of coronary heart disease, cancer, osteoporosis, obesity and tooth decay.

Unfortunately, many people feel that they do not have the resources or the information necessary to improve their own diet, and believe that healthy eating is all to do with prohibitions, restrictions and food supplements. Nothing could be further from the truth. Naturopathic nutrition makes it possible for everyone to enjoy a healthy diet – without calorie counting, complicated dietary reference tables, food supplements or painful self-denial – because it is based on one simple fact: **If you meet your daily energy needs with healthy foods, you will automatically get all the essential nutrients you need for good health.**

Part One made it clear that *You Are What You Eat* is not about restricting choice. It is about choosing to eat more of the huge variety of inexpensive foods that are good for you. It does not recommend rare or expensive ingredients or complicated combinations of food-supplement pills. Applying the ten Personal Eating Principles on a day-to-day basis is simply a matter of paying attention to what you eat, when you eat, how you eat and where you eat. In other words:

1. There is no doubt that unadulterated plant-based foods are healthy for humans. So making sure that you eat plenty of these simple, natural food-stuffs each day will automatically leave less space for unhealthy foods.

2. Your digestive system only operates properly when you are relaxed. So trying to eat only at times when you are not angry, frustrated, stressed or in a hurry will automatically improve your digestion.

3. You already have a highly sophisticated built-in calorie counter – your appetite – so you can easily adjust the amount you eat to match your energy needs as long as you pay attention to what your appetite is telling you. Many of us are so busy doing or thinking something else when we eat that we forget to chew, taste and enjoy our food. Making the process of eating a pleasurable and interesting experience makes it easier to notice when our appetite is saying 'more' or 'enough'.

4. Your ability to enjoy food relates very much to where you are eating. So it is important to choose the best environment you can find – according to your particular circumstances – in which to take your meals.

Here then, is a simple six-step guide to putting the Personal Eating Principles into practice. Whether you are a meat eater (omnivore), an eggs-cheese-and-milk vegetarian (lacto-ovo vegetarian) or eat no foods of animal origin (one hundred percent vegetarian), following this method will help you to create a diet for yourself which is:

- high in fibre and complex carbohydrate;
- high in polyunsaturates and essential fatty acids;
- high in natural anti-oxidants like vitamin E, vitamin C and vitamin A;
- rich in all important minerals including calcium, magnesium, iron and trace elements such as selenium;
- a good source of B vitamins;
- a rich and balanced source of protein and essential amino acids.

It will also be

- low in fat;
- low in saturates;
- low in cholesterol;
- low in hydrogenated fats and trans fats;

- low in refined sugar;
- free from harmful artificial additives.

Six-step guide

Step One

Complete a seven-day diet diary and analyse it according to the instructions in Chapter Six.

Step Two

On pages 46–53 you will find two Comparison Charts – one for males, the other for females – to help you compare your diet with a healthy diet based on the ten Personal Eating Principles. Choose the chart that applies to you and fill in the boxes in the *Your Diet* column with the number of portions you ate of the different food groups, as recorded in your Weekly Portion Totals list on pages 37–40.

Step Three

Compare the numbers you have recorded in the *Your Diet* column with the numbers printed in the *Recommended* column for your type of diet. Then, for each food group in turn, subtract the smaller number from the larger number and write the result in the *Difference* column, adding a plus (+) sign if you are eating more than the recommended amount and a minus (−) sign if you are eating less. You will end up with a chart looking something like the one featured overleaf.

Step Four

Using the *Difference* column as a guide, adjust your diet so that, in any one week, you eat the recommended number of helpings from **all** the recommended food groups for your type of diet[1]. What you eat on any particular day and how you combine the various recommended foods is entirely up to you. The system is flexible according to your taste, need and pocket. Eat the recommended number of helpings from the recommended food groups

---

[1] It may take a few weeks to get used to this new way of eating, so don't worry if you eat a few helpings more or less than recommended at first.

Food Group	Your Diet	Weekly Portion Totals			Male Difference
		Recommended			
		100% vegetarian	lacto-ovo vegetarian	omni-vore	
1. Roots and Tubers					
1a. Beetroot, carrot, etc.	4	10	10	10	−6
1b. Potatoes, etc.	7	5	5	5	+2
1c. Ginger	0	*	*	*	
1d. Horseradish	0	*	*	*	
1e. Radishes	2	*	*	*	
2. Bulbs					
2a. Onions, etc.	10	7	7	7	+3
2b. Garlic	1	3	3	3	−2
3. Stems					
3a. Celery, fennel	5	3	3	3	+2

over the week as a whole and you will automatically eat according to the first six Personal Eating Principles. The size of the helpings is up to you. Unless you are worried about your weight or fall into a special need category (see Chapter Eight), meeting your weekly energy requirements simply involves letting your appetite decide when you should eat more and when you have had enough. If you practise listening to your appetite, you will start to regulate your food-helping sizes to match your needs without thinking. You may even find that you are eating larger portions than previously of certain foods, but this is quite normal. Healthy foods are often lower in calories weight-for-weight, so you may need to eat more of them to get your full quota of energy.

Step Five

Read through Personal Eating Principles 7 to 10 again on pages 14–15. Decide if there are any practical ways in which you could alter your shopping habits to improve the quality of the food you buy, and act accordingly. Then decide whether it would be possible to increase the time and space

you allow during the day for cooking, eating, enjoying and digesting food –
and put your decisions into practice.

Step Six

To help you during your first week or so of eating healthily, use the Weekly
Running Total Chart at the end of this chapter (pages 55–61) to help you
keep track of your weekly intake of recommended foods.

Within just a few weeks, you will find that your new approach to eating
becomes an enjoyable habit, and that you are naturally choosing to eat more
of the foods that make you healthy and less of those that do you harm. The
more you choose to eat foods from the recommended food groups, the
healthier your diet will become. The more energy you get from natural low-
fat, low-sugar foods, the less room there will be for artificial high-fat, high-
sugar products. Eat what you feel your body needs of healthy foods and you
will provide your body with all the essential nutrients it needs to be well.

In Chapter Eight you will find answers to twenty common questions
about improving your diet which you also may find helpful. Since naturopathic nutrition usually means adding new foods to the weekly menu and
experiencing new tastes and textures, you might also like to try some of the
recipes in Chapters Twelve and Thirteen which show how a wider variety of
plant-based foods in your diet can be both tasty and nutritious.

COMPARISON CHART – Male

1. For the full list of foods in each food group, see pages 55–61
2. For details of possible substitutions between different food groups, see page 54

Key: 0 = Not part of your diet
      x = Not recommended
      * = No set recommendation

Food Group	Your Diet	Weekly Portion Totals Recommended			Male Difference
		100% vegetarian	lacto-ovo vegetarian	omni-vore	
1. Roots and Tubers					
1a. Beetroot, carrot, etc.		10	10	10	
1b. Potatoes, etc.		5	5	5	
1c. Ginger		*	*	*	
1d. Horseradish		*	*	*	
1e. Radishes		*	*	*	
2. Bulbs					
2a. Onions, etc.		7	7	7	
2b. Garlic		3	3	3	
3. Stems					
3a. Celery, fennel		3	3	3	
4. Leaves					
4a. Greens		8	8	8	
4b. Salads		7	7	7	
4c. Cress		2	2	2	
4d. Herbs		10	10	10	
5. Flowers					
5a. Artichokes, etc.		4	4	4	
6. Seeds					
6a. Pulses					
i) Fresh pulses		5	5	5	

Food Group	Your Diet	Weekly Portion Totals			Male Difference
		Recommended			
		100% vegetarian	lacto-ovo vegetarian	omni-vore	
6a. Pulses, cont.					
ii) Sprouts	☐	3	3	3	☐
iii) Dried pulses (VS)	☐	3	0	0	☐
iv) Lentils (VS)	☐	3	0	0	☐
v) Soya products (VS)	☐	3	0	0	☐
vi) Soya milk	☐	7	0	0	☐
vii) Baked beans	☐	*	*	*	☐
viii) Hummus (VS)	☐	1	0	0	☐
6b. Grains					
i) Wholegrains, flours	☐	5	5	5	☐
ii) Rice products	☐	6	6	6	☐
iii) Breads	☐	21	21	21	☐
iv) Pasta	☐	3	3	3	☐
v) Sugar-free cereals	☐	7	7	7	☐
vi) Other cereals	☐	X	X	X	☐
vii) Misc. grain products	☐	*	*	*	☐
6c. Spices	☐	5	5	5	☐
6d. Nuts and seeds					
i) Almonds, etc. (VS)	☐	5	0	0	☐
ii) Coconut	☐	X	X	X	☐
7. Fruits					
7a. Vegetable fruits					
i) Aubergine, etc.	☐	12	12	12	☐
ii) Avocados	☐	1	1	1	☐
iii) Okra	☐	*	*	*	☐
iv) Olives	☐	*	*	*	☐

Food Group	Your Diet	Weekly Portion Totals Recommended			Male Difference
		100% vegetarian	lacto-ovo vegetarian	omni-vore	
7b. Sweet fruits					
i) Apples and pears	☐	7	7	7	☐
ii) Melons	☐	3	3	3	☐
iii) Tropical fruits	☐	5	5	5	☐
iv) Soft fruits	☐	5	5	5	☐
7c. Citrus fruits	☐	5	5	5	☐
7d. Dried fruits	☐	5	5	5	☐
8. Berries					
8a. Blackberries, etc.	☐	4	4	4	☐
9. Fungi					
9a. All types of mushroom	☐	5	5	5	☐
10. Oils					
10a. Oils high in saturates	☐	X	X	X	☐
10b. Oils high in mono-us. (VS)	☐	7	0	0	☐
10c. Oils high in polyunsats.	☐	7	7	7	☐
10d. Polyunsat. margarines	☐	21	0	0	☐
10e. Other margarines	☐	X	X	X	☐
11. Miscellaneous Plant Products					
11a. Yeast extracts	☐	14	14	14	☐
11b. Soya sauce	☐	5	5	5	☐
11c. Vinegar	☐	5	5	5	☐
11d. Seaweeds	☐	2	2	2	☐
12. Dairy					
12a. Milk and milk products					
i) Cheese (DS)	☐	0	7	2	☐
ii) Cottage cheese (DS)	☐	0	5	0	☐

| Food Group | Your Diet | Weekly Portion Totals | | | Male Difference |
| | | Recommended | | | |
		100% vegetarian	lacto-ovo vegetarian	omni-vore	
12a. Milk products, cont.					
iii) Cream cheese (DS)		0	5	0	
iv) Low-fat yoghurt (DS)		0	5	0	
v) Semi-skim milk		0	7	7	
vi) Butter		0	21	21	
12b. Eggs		0	5	1	
13. Meats					
13a. Meat		0	0	2	
13b. Fowl		0	0	2	
13c. Processed meat, offal		0	0	1	
14. Fish					
14a. Lean fish (FS)		0	0	1	
14b. Oily fish (FS)		0	0	1	
14c. Shellfish (FS)		0	0	1	
15. Drinks					
15a. Water		ad lib	ad lib	ad lib	
15b. Pure fruit juice		7	7	7	
15c. Soft drinks and mixers		X	X	X	
15d. Caffeinated beverages		X	X	X	
15e. Caffeine-free beverages		*	*	*	
16. Sweet Foods and Snacks					
16a. Confectionery		X	X	X	
16b. Sugar, syrups, spreads		X	X	X	
16c. Cakes and biscuits		X	X	X	
16d. Savoury snacks		X	X	X	

COMPARISON CHART – Female

1. For the full list of foods in each food group, see pages 55–61
2. For details of possible substitutions between different food groups, see page 54

Key: 0 = Not part of your diet
       x = Not recommended
       * = No set recommendation

Food Group	Your Diet	Weekly Portion Totals Recommended			Female Difference
		100% vegetarian	lacto-ovo vegetarian	omni-vore	
1. Roots and Tubers					
1a. Beetroot, carrot, etc.		6	6	6	
1b. Potatoes, etc.		3	3	3	
1c. Ginger		*	*	*	
1d. Horseradish		*	*	*	
1e. Radishes		*	*	*	
2. Bulbs					
2a. Onions, etc.		5	5	5	
2b. Garlic		3	3	3	
3. Stems					
3a. Celery, fennel		3	3	3	
4. Leaves					
4a. Greens		6	6	6	
4b. Salads		5	5	5	
4c. Cress		2	2	2	
4d. Herbs		10	10	10	
5. Flowers					
5a. Artichokes, etc.		4	4	4	
6. Seeds					
6a. Pulses					
i) Fresh pulses		4	4	4	

| Food Group | Your Diet | Weekly Portion Totals | | | Female Difference |
| | | Recommended | | | |
		100% vegetarian	lacto-ovo vegetarian	omni-vore	
6a. Pulses, cont.					
ii) Sprouts		2	2	2	
iii) Dried pulses (VS)		2	0	0	
iv) Lentils (VS)		2	0	0	
v) Soya products (VS)		2	0	0	
vi) Soya milk		7	0	0	
vii) Baked beans		*	*	*	
viii) Hummus (VS)		1	0	0	
6b. Grains					
i) Wholegrains, flours		3	3	3	
ii) Rice products		4	4	4	
iii) Breads		14	14	14	
iv) Pasta		2	2	2	
v) Sugar-free cereals		7	7	7	
vi) Other cereals		X	X	X	
vii) Misc. grain products		*	*	*	
6c. Spices		5	5	5	
6d. Nuts and seeds					
i) Almonds, etc. (VS)		3	0	0	
ii) Coconut		X	X	X	
7. Fruits					
7a. Vegetable fruits					
i) Aubergine, etc.		8	8	8	
ii) Avocados		1	1	1	
iii) Okra		*	*	*	
iv) Olives		*	*	*	

Food Group	Your Diet	Weekly Portion Totals			Female Difference
		Recommended			
		100% vegetarian	lacto-ovo vegetarian	omni-vore	
7b. Sweet fruits					
i) Apples and pears		5	5	5	
ii) Melons		1	1	1	
iii) Tropical fruits		5	5	5	
iv) Soft fruits		5	5	5	
7c. Citrus fruits		5	5	5	
7d. Dried fruits		5	5	5	
8. Berries					
8a. Blackberries, etc.		4	4	4	
9. Fungi					
9a. All types of mushroom		3	3	3	
10. Oils					
10a. Oils high in saturates		X	X	X	
10b. Oils high in mono-us. (VS)		5	0	0	
10c. Oils high in polyunsats.		5	5	5	
10d. Polyunsat. margarines		14	0	0	
10e. Other margarines		X	X	X	
11. Miscellaneous Plant Products					
11a. Yeast extracts		14	14	14	
11b. Soya sauce		5	5	5	
11c. Vinegar		2	2	2	
11d. Seaweed		2	2	2	
12. Dairy					
12a. Milk and milk products					
i) Cheese (DS)		0	5	2	
ii) Cottage cheese (DS)		0	3	0	

Food Group	Your Diet	Weekly Portion Totals Recommended			Female Difference
		100% vegetarian	lacto-ovo vegetarian	omni-vore	
12a. Milk products, cont.					
iii) Cream cheese (DS)		0	3	0	
iv) Low-fat yoghurt (DS)		0	3	0	
v) Semi-skim milk		0	7	7	
vi) Butter		0	14	14	
12b. Eggs		0	3	1	
13. Meats					
13a. Meat		0	0	1	
13b. Fowl		0	0	1	
13c. Processed meat, offal		0	0	1	
14. Fish					
14a. Lean fish (FS)		0	0	1	
14b. Oily fish (FS)		0	0	0	
14c. Shellfish (FS)		0	0	1	
15. Drinks					
15a. Water		ad lib	ad lib	ad lib	
15b. Pure fruit juice		7	7	7	
15c. Soft drinks and mixers		X	X	X	
15d. Caffeinated beverages		X	X	X	
15e. Caffeine-free beverages		*	*	*	
16. Sweet Foods and Snacks					
16a. Confectionery		X	X	X	
16b. Sugar, syrups, spreads		X	X	X	
16c. Cakes and biscuits		X	X	X	
16d. Savoury snacks		X	X	X	

Substitutions

If you are an omnivore, but would like to eat less meat and more fish and/or dairy products and/or vegetable foods, you can choose to make the following portion substitutions.

Each portion of meat (Group 13) can be swapped for:

One portion of fish (those marked FS in group 14)
or
Three modest portions of dairy products (those marked DS in group 12)
or
Two generous portions of vegetable foods (those marked VS in groups 6 and 10).

If you would like to cut down on butter, you can swap portion for portion with polyunsaturated margarine. If you would like to cut down on cow's milk, you can swap portion for portion with soya milk.

If you would like to eat less dairy products and more vegetable foods, you can make the following substitutions:

Portions of dairy products marked DS in group 12 can be swapped one for one with portions of vegetable foods marked VS in groups 6 and 10.

Weekly running total chart

Instructions

1. Fill in the blank Target boxes in the following Weekly Running Total Chart with the recommended number of helpings for each food group, as given in the Comparison Chart for your particular type of diet. You may find it best to photocopy the chart before filling it in.

2. Carry the Weekly Running Total Chart with you during your first week of diet adjustment. Cross off numbers (in pencil) every time you eat a helping of food from any of your recommended food groups.

3. Use the chart to make sure that by the end of the week you have eaten approximately the recommended number of helpings from each recommended food group.

You may find the following meal plan helpful to get you started:

    A. *Breakfast* Fresh fruits and grains (such as muesli or porridge)
    B. *Lunch* Main meal with plenty of fresh vegetables
    C. *Supper* Salad meal including some raw food.

B and C can be swapped to suit your daily routine.

4. Repeat the exercise as necessary, until you feel quite familiar with your new diet.

WEEKLY RUNNING TOTAL CHART

1. Roots and Tubers

1a. Beetroot, carrot, celeriac, parsnip, swede, turnip   **Target** ☐

    1 2 3 4 5 6 7 8 9 10 11 12 13 14 15 16 17 18 19 20 21 22 23 24 25

1b. All potatoes, sweet potatoes, yams   **Target** ☐

    1 2 3 4 5 6 7 8 9 10 11 12 13 14 15 16 17 18 19 20 21 22 23 24 25

1c. Ginger   **Target** ☐

    1 2 3 4 5 6 7 8 9 10 11 12 13 14 15 16 17 18 19 20 21 22 23 24 25

1d. Horseradish   **Target** ☐

    1 2 3 4 5 6 7 8 9 10 11 12 13 14 15 16 17 18 19 20 21 22 23 24 25

1e. Radishes   **Target** ☐

    1 2 3 4 5 6 7 8 9 10 11 12 13 14 15 16 17 18 19 20 21 22 23 24 25

2. Bulbs

2a. Onions, shallots, spring onions, leeks   **Target** ☐

    1 2 3 4 5 6 7 8 9 10 11 12 13 14 15 16 17 18 19 20 21 22 23 24 25

2b. Garlic   **Target** ☐

    1 2 3 4 5 6 7 8 9 10 11 12 13 14 15 16 17 18 19 20 21 22 23 24 25

3. Stems

3a. Celery, fennel   **Target** ☐

    1 2 3 4 5 6 7 8 9 10 11 12 13 14 15 16 17 18 19 20 21 22 23 24 25

WEEKLY RUNNING TOTAL CHART, *continued*

4. Leaves

4a. Greens (brussels sprouts, cabbage, curly kale, endive, spinach, spring greens)   **Target** [ ]

1 2 3 4 5 6 7 8 9 10 11 12 13 14 15 16 17 18 19 20 21 22 23 24 25

4b. Salads (all lettuces)   **Target** [ ]

1 2 3 4 5 6 7 8 9 10 11 12 13 14 15 16 17 18 19 20 21 22 23 24 25

4c. Cress (mustard and cress, watercress)   **Target** [ ]

1 2 3 4 5 6 7 8 9 10 11 12 13 14 15 16 17 18 19 20 21 22 23 24 25

4d. Herbs (basil, chives, coriander, dill, mint, oregano, parsley, rosemary, sage, tarragon, thyme)   **Target** [ ]

1 2 3 4 5 6 7 8 9 10 11 12 13 14 15 16 17 18 19 20 21 22 23 24 25

5. Flowers

5a. Artichoke, asparagus, cauliflower, green broccoli, purple broccoli   **Target** [ ]

1 2 3 4 5 6 7 8 9 10 11 12 13 14 15 16 17 18 19 20 21 22 23 24 25

6. Seeds

6a. Pulses

   i) Fresh Pulses (broad beans, green beans, runner beans, mange tout, all peas)   **Target** [ ]

1 2 3 4 5 6 7 8 9 10 11 12 13 14 15 16 17 18 19 20 21 22 23 24 25

   ii) Sprouts   **Target** [ ]

1 2 3 4 5 6 7 8 9 10 11 12 13 14 15 16 17 18 19 20 21 22 23 24 25

   iii) Dried Pulses (aduki beans, black gram, blackeye beans, butter beans, chick-peas, etc.)   **Target** [ ]

1 2 3 4 5 6 7 8 9 10 11 12 13 14 15 16 17 18 19 20 21 22 23 24 25

   iv) Lentils (red, green, brown, dal, etc.)   **Target** [ ]

1 2 3 4 5 6 7 8 9 10 11 12 13 14 15 16 17 18 19 20 21 22 23 24 25

   v) Soya products (soya beans, tempeh, tofu)   **Target** [ ]

1 2 3 4 5 6 7 8 9 10 11 12 13 14 15 16 17 18 19 20 21 22 23 24 25

WEEKLY RUNNING TOTAL CHART, *continued*

6a. Pulses, cont.

vi) Soya milk   **Target** [   ]

1 2 3 4 5 6 7 8 9 10 11 12 13 14 15 16 17 18 19 20 21 22 23 24 25

vii) Baked beans   **Target** [   ]

1 2 3 4 5 6 7 8 9 10 11 12 13 14 15 16 17 18 19 20 21 22 23 24 25

viii) Hummus   **Target** [   ]

1 2 3 4 5 6 7 8 9 10 11 12 13 14 15 16 17 18 19 20 21 22 23 24 25

6b. Grains

i) Wholegrains and flours (barley, buckwheat, bulgur, couscous, millet, rye, wheat)   **Target** [   ]

1 2 3 4 5 6 7 8 9 10 11 12 13 14 15 16 17 18 19 20 21 22 23 24 25

ii) Rice products (brown rice, white rice, basmati, rice flour)   **Target** [   ]

1 2 3 4 5 6 7 8 9 10 11 12 13 14 15 16 17 18 19 20 21 22 23 24 25

iii) Breads (brown, white, wholemeal, rye)   **Target** [   ]

1 2 3 4 5 6 7 8 9 10 11 12 13 14 15 16 17 18 19 20 21 22 23 24 25 26
27 28 29 30 31 32 33 34 35 36 37 38 39 40 41 42 43 44 45 46 47 48

iv) Pasta (macaroni, spaghetti, tagliatelle, etc.)   **Target** [   ]

1 2 3 4 5 6 7 8 9 10 11 12 13 14 15 16 17 18 19 20 21 22 23 24 25

v) Sugar-free breakfast cereals (sugar-free muesli, porridge)   **Target** [   ]

1 2 3 4 5 6 7 8 9 10 11 12 13 14 15 16 17 18 19 20 21 22 23 24 25

vi) Other breakfast cereals   **Target** [   ]

1 2 3 4 5 6 7 8 9 10 11 12 13 14 15 16 17 18 19 20 21 22 23 24 25

vii) Miscellaneous grain products (bran, cornflour, oatmeal, oatcakes, sago, semolina, sweetcorn, wheatgerm, etc.)   **Target** [   ]

1 2 3 4 5 6 7 8 9 10 11 12 13 14 15 16 17 18 19 20 21 22 23 24 25

WEEKLY RUNNING TOTAL CHART, *continued*

6c. Spices

  i) Anise, caraway, celery seed, coriander, cumin, dill,
     fennel, mustard, etc.   **Target** [   ]
     1 2 3 4 5 6 7 8 9 10 11 12 13 14 15 16 17 18 19 20 21 22 23 24 25

6d. Nuts and seeds

  i) Almonds, brazils, cashews, hazels, peanuts, pecans,
     pine kernels, pumpkin seeds, sesame seeds, sunflower
     seeds, walnuts (including nut butters)   **Target** [   ]
     1 2 3 4 5 6 7 8 9 10 11 12 13 14 15 16 17 18 19 20 21 22 23 24 25

  ii) Coconut   **Target** [   ]
     1 2 3 4 5 6 7 8 9 10 11 12 13 14 15 16 17 18 19 20 21 22 23 24 25

7. Fruits

7a. Vegetable fruits

  i) Aubergine, courgette, cucumber, marrow, pepper,
     pumpkin, squash, tomato   **Target** [   ]
     1 2 3 4 5 6 7 8 9 10 11 12 13 14 15 16 17 18 19 20 21 22 23 24 25

  ii) Avocado   **Target** [   ]
     1 2 3 4 5 6 7 8 9 10 11 12 13 14 15 16 17 18 19 20 21 22 23 24 25

  iii) Okra   **Target** [   ]
     1 2 3 4 5 6 7 8 9 10 11 12 13 14 15 16 17 18 19 20 21 22 23 24 25

  iv) Olives   **Target** [   ]
     1 2 3 4 5 6 7 8 9 10 11 12 13 14 15 16 17 18 19 20 21 22 23 24 25

7b. Sweet fruits

  i) Apples and pears (all types)   **Target** [   ]
     1 2 3 4 5 6 7 8 9 10 11 12 13 14 15 16 17 18 19 20 21 22 23 24 25

  ii) Melons (all types)   **Target** [   ]
     1 2 3 4 5 6 7 8 9 10 11 12 13 14 15 16 17 18 19 20 21 22 23 24 25

  iii) Tropical fruits (mango, pawpaw, banana, passion, pineapple) **Target** [   ]
     1 2 3 4 5 6 7 8 9 10 11 12 13 14 15 16 17 18 19 20 21 22 23 24 25

WEEKLY RUNNING TOTAL CHART, *continued*

7b. Sweet fruits, cont.

iv) Soft fruits (apricots, peaches, plums, nectarines,
sharon fruit, grapes, cherries) **Target** [   ]

1 2 3 4 5 6 7 8 9 10 11 12 13 14 15 16 17 18 19 20 21 22 23 24 25

7c. Citrus fruits (clementine, grapefruit, lemon, orange,
satsuma, tangerine) **Target** [   ]

1 2 3 4 5 6 7 8 9 10 11 12 13 14 15 16 17 18 19 20 21 22 23 24 25

7d. Dried fruits (apricots, dates, figs, prunes, raisins, sultanas, etc.) **Target** [   ]

1 2 3 4 5 6 7 8 9 10 11 12 13 14 15 16 17 18 19 20 21 22 23 24 25

8. Berries

8a. Blackberries, blackcurrants, cranberries, gooseberries,
raspberries, redcurrants, strawberries **Target** [   ]

1 2 3 4 5 6 7 8 9 10 11 12 13 14 15 16 17 18 19 20 21 22 23 24 25

9. Fungi

9a. All types of mushroom **Target** [   ]

1 2 3 4 5 6 7 8 9 10 11 12 13 14 15 16 17 18 19 20 21 22 23 24 25

10. Oils

10a. Oils high in saturates (coconut, palm, animal fats and oils) **Target** [   ]

1 2 3 4 5 6 7 8 9 10 11 12 13 14 15 16 17 18 19 20 21 22 23 24 25

10b. Oils high in mono-unsaturates (hazelnut, olive, peanut) **Target** [   ]

1 2 3 4 5 6 7 8 9 10 11 12 13 14 15 16 17 18 19 20 21 22 23 24 25

10c. Oils high in polyunsaturates (corn, evening primrose,
grapeseed, safflower, sesame, soya, sunflower,
vegetable, walnut, wheatgerm) **Target** [   ]

1 2 3 4 5 6 7 8 9 10 11 12 13 14 15 16 17 18 19 20 21 22 23 24 25

10d. Polyunsaturated margarines (containing no
hydrogenated fats) **Target** [   ]

1 2 3 4 5 6 7 8 9 10 11 12 13 14 15 16 17 18 19 20 21 22 23 24 25

10e. Other margarines **Target** [   ]

1 2 3 4 5 6 7 8 9 10 11 12 13 14 15 16 17 18 19 20 21 22 23 24 25

WEEKLY RUNNING TOTAL CHART, *continued*

11. Miscellaneous Plant Products

11a. Yeast extracts (eg. Marmite)   **Target** [   ]

1 2 3 4 5 6 7 8 9 10 11 12 13 14 15 16 17 18 19 20 21 22 23 24 25

11b. Soya sauce   **Target** [   ]

1 2 3 4 5 6 7 8 9 10 11 12 13 14 15 16 17 18 19 20 21 22 23 24 25

11c. Vinegar   **Target** [   ]

1 2 3 4 5 6 7 8 9 10 11 12 13 14 15 16 17 18 19 20 21 22 23 24 25

11d. Seaweeds   **Target** [   ]

1 2 3 4 5 6 7 8 9 10 11 12 13 14 15 16 17 18 19 20 21 22 23 24 25

12. Dairy

12a. Milk and milk products (all types of cow, goat and
sheep milk, cheese and yoghurt)   **Target** [   ]

1 2 3 4 5 6 7 8 9 10 11 12 13 14 15 16 17 18 19 20 21 22 23 24 25

12b. Eggs (all types)   **Target** [   ]

1 2 3 4 5 6 7 8 9 10 11 12 13 14 15 16 17 18 19 20 21 22 23 24 25

13. Meats

13a. Meat (beef, lamb, pork, venison, etc.)   **Target** [   ]

1 2 3 4 5 6 7 8 9 10 11 12 13 14 15 16 17 18 19 20 21 22 23 24 25

13b. Fowl (chicken, duck, game birds, goose, turkey)   **Target** [   ]

1 2 3 4 5 6 7 8 9 10 11 12 13 14 15 16 17 18 19 20 21 22 23 24 25

13c. Processed meat and offal (all dried, cured and processed
meats – ham, salami, sausages, meat pies, etc. – plus all
offal products, ie. brawn, heart, liver, kidney, etc.)   **Target** [   ]

1 2 3 4 5 6 7 8 9 10 11 12 13 14 15 16 17 18 19 20 21 22 23 24 25

14. Fish

14a. Lean fish (cod, plaice, whiting, sole, etc.)   **Target** [   ]

1 2 3 4 5 6 7 8 9 10 11 12 13 14 15 16 17 18 19 20 21 22 23 24 25

WEEKLY RUNNING TOTAL CHART, *continued*

14b. Oily fish (herring, mackerel, salmon, etc.)   **Target** [   ]
    1 2 3 4 5 6 7 8 9 10 11 12 13 14 15 16 17 18 19 20 21 22 23 24 25

14c. Shellfish (all types)   **Target** [   ]
    1 2 3 4 5 6 7 8 9 10 11 12 13 14 15 16 17 18 19 20 21 22 23 24 25

15. Drinks
15a. Water   **Target** [   ]
    1 2 3 4 5 6 7 8 9 10 11 12 13 14 15 16 17 18 19 20 21 22 23 24 25

15b. Pure fruit juice   **Target** [   ]
    1 2 3 4 5 6 7 8 9 10 11 12 13 14 15 16 17 18 19 20 21 22 23 24 25

15c. Soft drinks and mixers   **Target** [   ]
    1 2 3 4 5 6 7 8 9 10 11 12 13 14 15 16 17 18 19 20 21 22 23 24 25

15d. Caffeinated beverages (tea, coffee, etc.)   **Target** [   ]
    1 2 3 4 5 6 7 8 9 10 11 12 13 14 15 16 17 18 19 20 21 22 23 24 25

15e. Caffeine-free beverages (herb teas, dandelion 'coffees',
    roast barley 'coffees', etc.)   **Target** [   ]
    1 2 3 4 5 6 7 8 9 10 11 12 13 14 15 16 17 18 19 20 21 22 23 24 25

16. Sweet Foods and Snacks
16a. All types of confectionery (sweets, chocolates, candies, etc.) **Target** [   ]
    1 2 3 4 5 6 7 8 9 10 11 12 13 14 15 16 17 18 19 20 21 22 23 24 25

16b. Sugar, syrups and spreads (sugar, cane syrup, maple
    syrup, jam, marmalade, honey)   **Target** [   ]
    1 2 3 4 5 6 7 8 9 10 11 12 13 14 15 16 17 18 19 20 21 22 23 24 25

16c. Cakes and biscuits (all types)   **Target** [   ]
    1 2 3 4 5 6 7 8 9 10 11 12 13 14 15 16 17 18 19 20 21 22 23 24 25

16d. Savoury snacks (crisps, etc.)   **Target** [   ]
    1 2 3 4 5 6 7 8 9 10 11 12 13 14 15 16 17 18 19 20 21 22 23 24 25

CHAPTER EIGHT

20 COMMON QUESTIONS ABOUT NATUROPATHIC NUTRITION

This chapter will give you detailed answers to the twenty most common questions people ask about naturopathic nutrition. We hope that it will provide you with the information you need to get the most out of your new way of eating.

Overview

1. How can I be sure of getting enough energy for my height, weight and activity level when I start eating more healthily?   page 63

2. Is white sugar really so bad for you?   page 64

3. What about coffee, tea and salt?   page 65

4. What is the best way to increase my fibre intake?   page 67

5. Does it matter if I can't get organic produce?   page 70

6. Is there such a thing as first and second class proteins?   page 72

7. How much protein do I need to eat to be healthy?   page 76

8. Saturated fats, hydrogenated fats, trans fats, cholesterol, unsaturated fats, essential fatty acids – what are they and are they OK to eat?   page 79

9. Should I be taking anti-oxidant supplements to protect against free radicals?   page 86

10. Is raw food better for health than cooked food?   page 87

11. How do I avoid suffering from wind?   page 88

12. If I choose not to eat any animal produce, won't I get deficient in some important vitamins?   page 89

13. Should I be taking calcium supplements to avoid osteoporosis? page 91

14. Is soya safe?   page 94

15. Can naturopathic nutrition help with weight loss?   page 96

16. What foods are good for weaning my baby on to solids?   page 100

17. How does naturopathic nutrition apply to childhood and adolescence? page 101

18. How should my diet change as I get older?   page 103

19. What special dietary precautions should I take during pregnancy? page 104

20. Why is breast feeding better than bottle feeding and should I be eating more if I am breast-feeding?   page 106

I. *How can I be sure of getting enough energy for my height, weight and activity level when I start eating more healthily?*

Nature has given your body a very efficient system for matching the energy you take in the form of food with the energy you use up by doing physical, mental and metabolic work: when you need energy, you feel hungry and when you've eaten enough, you feel full. Simple as it is, this system is all most of us need to make sure that we eat the right number of calories for our particular energy needs each day.

Of course, big people tend to need more calories than small people, and on average men require more calories than women to remain healthy. On the whole, however, we do not need to carry around calculators and calorie charts to get our calorie intake right. If we eat healthy foods, our bodies already know how to do the calorie calculations. All we have to do is eat when we are hungry and stop eating when we are satisfied.

That is why the recommended numbers of portions given in the last chapter apply to nearly everyone (except children and others with particular needs – see below), regardless of their size or sex. In general, small people do not eat less helpings of food per week than big people; they simply adjust their portion sizes to suit their energy needs. In other words, meeting your weekly energy requirements simply involves letting your appetite decide when to eat and when you have had enough. If you eat enough of the recommended foods each week to fulfil your energy needs, you will automatically eat all you need of all essential nutrients.

If you are particularly active, either in your leisure time or at work, remember that it is perfectly normal and desirable to eat more than people who are less active. Adolescents and women who are pregnant or breast feeding also tend to eat more to meet their increased energy requirements (see questions 17, 19 and 20, pages 101, 104 and 106). Older people, on the other hand, tend to require less energy from their food as life becomes less active (see question 18, page 103).

Athletes – especially those involved in competitive sports – should be aware that heavy training schedules can greatly increase their energy needs, and they should therefore seek specialist advice on diet. Unfortunately, they are sometimes prey to the aggressive marketing of a variety of nutritional supplements, few (if any) of which have been reliably shown to boost performance. On the other hand, several world class athletes achieve and maintain their levels of fitness and performance simply by following a diet based on fruits, grains, nuts and vegetables.

To sum up, the human race has thrived for hundreds of thousands of years, without scientists or nutrition tables, by using nature's own system of food intake control – appetite. Listen to your appetite and you will eat enough calories. Eat enough calories and you will meet your energy needs. Meet your energy needs with healthy foods and you will get all the essential nutrients you need for good health.

2. Is white sugar really so bad for you?

To most people, 'sugar' is a packet of small, sweet-tasting white or brown crystals bought from a shop. In fact, food contains at least seventeen different types of sugar, all slightly different and all part of the carbohydrate family. (Carbohydrates – sugars and starches – are made by plants out of air and sunlight, and are the main source of energy in human diets. They are essential to health and are discussed in more detail in Chapter Four.)

Not all the sugar we eat is good for us and, in recent years, the health spotlight has been turned on one particular type of sugar – refined sucrose – a substance which some have labelled 'pure, white and deadly'. However, since the average Westerner consumes about 30kg of refined sugar per year, the idea that sugar is bad for you is hotly disputed by the sugar industry. The truth is that sugar packaged naturally within foods such as fruits and vegetables is a normal and useful part of the human diet; but sucrose *extracted* from sugar cane or sugar-beet and *added* to other foods is a health hazard.

Until about one hundred years ago, sugar was an expensive delicacy and was only available as an occasional treat. These days, a glance at supermarket food labels shows refined sugar turning up all over the place, often in processed foods that also contain high levels of fat.

Eating refined sugar causes tooth decay and obesity, both of which are serious health problems in Western society. Scientists around the world have also made links between refined sugar consumption and a whole range of diseases including late-onset diabetes, heart disease, Crohn's disease, gall-stones, candida and cancers, such as breast and bowel cancer.

To make matters worse, the more refined sugar we eat, the less likely we are to be eating proper amounts of other nutrients. Although sugar quickly satisfies hunger, it contains no vitamins, minerals[1], proteins, fats or fibre, and the short burst of energy it provides is usually followed by a bout of extreme tiredness which we tend to overcome with another sugar fix. These episodes of tiredness can become such a feature of daily life that our overall activity level drops and we then risk gaining weight because of eating more calories than we need.

Of course, sugar is not bad in itself. Used in small amounts as a condiment – like salt and pepper – it can certainly add interest to our diet. But eating sugar taken out of its normal context and concentrated into processed food in anything but small amounts is bad for health, and we would do well to avoid it wherever possible. With over seventy percent of available food now being processed in one way or another, and with sugar being added to so much processed food, eating whole foods becomes an ever-more attractive option.

3. *What about coffee, tea and salt?*

If coffee were regarded as a drug, not a beverage, it would probably be described rather like this:

> Coffee is a pharmacological agent which, at low doses, increases alertness by increasing the rate of energy usage in the body. In high doses, it can be toxic, producing a variety of symptoms including increased heart rate and nervousness. There is no completely convincing direct evidence of harmful side effects, but it is associated with an increased risk of

[1] Raw cane sugar does contain small amounts of iron and B vitamins, but has no other health advantages over other refined sugars.

developing bladder cancer. It is also known to bring on migraine in susceptible people. There are suggestions that coffee, especially when prepared by boiling, may increase blood cholesterol levels; many people also report that coffee exaggerates the symptoms of stomach ulcers and hiatus hernia. There has been unsubstantiated research indicating that coffee may be protective against cancer of the colon and rectum.

Tea has the same basic effects of increasing alertness in low doses and causing nervousness in high doses, but there is no mainstream scientific evidence that tea drinking is definitely associated with disease. So, at first sight, it is not easy to see why so much healthy diet advice includes the recommendation to reduce or cut out coffee and tea.

The reasons for the unpopularity of coffee and tea amongst advocates of a healthier lifestyle are twofold. Firstly, with so many people suffering from the effects of stress and overstimulation in the late 1990s, it is illogical voluntarily to take substances that stimulate us more and, at the same time, make us use up our available energy more quickly. In other words, although caffeine-containing drinks (including many popular soft drinks) may stimulate us in the short term, the cost is that we feel more tired, more quickly, in the long term.

Secondly, it is the common experience of practitioners of many different medical disciplines that people suffering from chronic illness – particularly arthritis and rheumatic complaints – often feel much better when they stop drinking tea and coffee. The many theories put forward to explain this effect are not generally accepted by orthodox scientists, but the phenomenon is easy to understand when you remember that, in all illness, it takes energy to get better. Any substance that causes us to use up energy more quickly than we would do otherwise (such as coffee) must therefore make it harder for us to recover from illness.

The benefits felt by those who give up stimulants like tea and coffee far outweigh the initial difficulty of changing an ingrained habit, although it may take several weeks for the sense of extra vitality and well-being to emerge. So if you do decide to alter your tea and coffee intake, give it a proper trial of at least six weeks before making your final decision. But beware: the toxic effects of tea and coffee – palpitations and nervousness – may take you by surprise if you drink a strong brew of either after a period of abstinence.

Common salt – sodium chloride – is a basic component of all animal bodies. Without it, our cells could not operate, and we would not be able to keep enough fluid in our bloodstream to function properly. Salt loss in sweat, faeces or urine caused by disease, injury or environmental stress may lead to life-threatening dehydration, and so our bodies have developed enormously complex and efficient salt management mechanisms.

In mankind's early history, salt was a rare commodity, thought so valuable that it was used as a trading 'currency'. Nowadays, it is so cheap and easy to obtain that we in the West routinely eat more than twenty times the amount we actually need each day. An appetite that once ensured that we got just enough salt to meet our basic needs has nowadays been transformed into a desire for stimulation of our taste buds. But does this really matter?

The debate about salt and health goes back fifty years or so, when it was first suggested that too much salt in the diet was linked to raised blood pressure. Since high blood pressure is a major contributing cause to our current Western epidemic of strokes and heart attacks, there has been much research into the topic, with the balance of opinion swaying back and forth over the years. Standing on the shoulders of past effort, modern research has now shown quite clearly that cutting down daily salt intake could significantly reduce the average blood pressure of the population, therefore saving tens of thousands of lives each year by reducing the occurrence of stroke and heart disease. However, only about fifteen percent of our average daily salt intake comes from added or table salt; eighty-five percent comes from food itself.

Table S1, over, shows two things clearly. Firstly, fresh, unprocessed foods contain very much less salt than processed foods. Secondly, most plant-based foods contain less salt than animal-based foods. So, the simplest way to reduce your daily salt intake is to reduce your consumption of processed foods and increase your intake of unprocessed plant-based foods. In other words, by following the advice in this book, you will naturally eat less salt.

4. *What is the best way to increase my fibre intake?*

Until the early 1950s, very few people were interested in dietary fibre. The 'indigestible' parts of plants (bits of the plant cell wall that resist the action of digestive juices) were thought to serve no useful function in the diet and they were therefore refined out of foodstuffs by manufacturers keen to produce pure, easy-to-digest products.

Nowadays, the label 'high fibre' is found on all sorts of foods, and most people in Western cultures are aware that there is some link between fibre and good health. Breakfast tables resound to the determined crunching of 'added bran' cereals, and it has become fashionable to leave the skins on potatoes, carrots and other vegetables.

Table S1 Salt content of some common foods

Unprocessed Foods	Mmol Sodium (as sodium chloride) per 100 grams
Wholemeal flour	0.1
Lettuce	0.4
Cabbage	0.3
Potatoes	0.3
Apples	0.1
Beef	3.0
Eggs	4.0
Milk	2.0
Cod	3.0
Processed Foods	
Bacon	81.0
Kippers	23.0
Salted butter	38.0
Cheddar cheese	27.0
Tomato ketchup	49.0
Baked beans	21.0

(Paul and Southgate)

There are three reasons for this turnaround in opinion. Firstly, there is good quality scientific evidence that a diet rich in natural fibre helps us to avoid a number of serious, common diseases, such as bowel cancer, diverticulitis, heart disease and gallstones.

Secondly, fibre affects the workings of the bowel and protects against constipation. This combination guarantees the interest of a huge audience, since many people have an abiding fascination for the workings of the southerly end of their digestive tracts, and are particularly keen to keep their 'motions' smooth and regular.

Thirdly, fibre is cheap. Adding fibre to a refined food product costs relatively little, but it enables food manufacturers to claim a 'health advantage'. It also adds weight and bulk to a product. These two features together add up to increased profit and so, where fibre is concerned, manufacturers have an incentive to make their products healthier. Of course, sugar and saturated fats are also cheap but, unfortunately for the consumer, adding more of these to foods makes them *less* healthy. Reducing fat and sugar in many food products would mean adding some more costly ingredients or increasing the price. Since most popular processed foods are sold in a highly competitive marketplace, food producers are loathe to do this. After all, brighter packaging, chemically enhanced flavours and inventive advertising are usually enough to maintain the sales of almost any food product, however poor its nutritional value.

In the late 1940s, two surgeons working in Africa (Dennis Burkitt and Hugh Trowell) noticed that there were considerable differences between the diseases suffered by the local population and by 'affluent' Westerners. In particular, they found that haemorrhoids, colorectal cancer, diverticular disease, appendicitis, coronary heart disease and gallstones were very rare amongst native Africans and constipation was almost unheard of. As a result of their observations, they coined the term 'diseases of civilization' to describe those diseases particularly associated with wealth and the Western lifestyle.

In 1953, a scientific paper by E H Hipsley defined dietary fibre as 'the material in food derived from plant cell walls' and, in 1960, Dr Trowell put forward the idea that fibre in the diet could be what protected sub-Saharan Africans from 'diseases of civilisation'. This speculation lead to a great deal of research into the effects of dietary fibre on human health and, as a result, the following is now known:

1. A diet low in fibre, but high in refined foods (ie. foods with the fibre more or less removed) causes hard, dry faeces, which pass slowly through the large intestine and require a lot of effort to get out.

2. Fibre in the diet increases the weight and bulk of the faeces and helps them pass through the large intestine more easily.

3. Fibre is not indigestible. Some of it is digested by the microbes that live in the large intestine. This process produces chemicals that are either used as food by the cells lining the inside of the large intestine or are absorbed into the blood and used to help regulate metabolism.

4. Not all fibre is the same. It is made up of a whole range of different plant materials (including cellulose and pectin), some of which dissolve in water (soluble fibre) and some of which do not (insoluble fibre). As a result, scientists nowadays tend to refer to fibre as Non-Starch Polysaccharides (NSPs), a blanket term covering all the different types.

5. Insoluble fibre (like wheat bran) increases the weight and bulk of faeces and protects against diseases like bowel cancer and diverticular disease. Soluble fibre (such as that found in fruits and vegetables) seems to protect against diseases associated with high blood cholesterol; for example, coronary heart disease and gallstones.

6. From the body's point of view, fibre contained in whole fruits and vegetables is much more useful than commercially processed 'added' fibre.

It is important to remember that Non-Starch Polysaccharides are *only* found in plant foods, particularly in vegetables. There are no NSPs in meat or dairy products. It is also important to do away with the idea that fibre is an indigestible waste product. The body uses fibre in several different ways depending on its type, what food it is in, how the food is prepared and on the individual nature of our digestions. Eating more fibre is not just a way of avoiding constipation – it also helps us to metabolize fats and sugars more effectively, and protects us from a variety of common, serious diseases.

Unfortunately, except for vegans and vegetarians, the average fibre intake of the Western population is so low that many people are constantly on the verge of constipation. On the other hand, it is widely agreed that even a quite modest increase in the amounts of fresh fruit, vegetables and wholemeal products we eat each day could have a significant effect on our health because, unlike most 'added fibre' products, fruits, vegetables and wholegrains provide us with all the NSPs we need in simple, cheap and tasty packages.

Note: You may have heard that eating too much fibre can interfere with your ability to absorb iron (and other minerals) from your diet, because some fibre-rich substances like wheat bran contain chemicals called phytates. This problem only arises when bran is extracted from cereals and then used to 'add fibre' to the diet. Apart from containing large quantities of iron, fruits and vegetables in their natural form contain vitamin C, which improves the absorption of iron from food. What is more, phytates in fruits and vegetables are known to protect against tooth decay.

5. *Does it matter if I can't get organic produce?*

Whatever sort of food you prefer, the naturopathic ideal is that it should be fresh, uncontaminated and locally grown or reared. It should also be cheap. Sadly, except for a lucky few with the land, time and space to grow their own food, meeting this ideal is virtually impossible for most of us in Western society.

We are told that an intensive farming system is necessary to ensure that we all have enough food at a cost low enough for every pocket. In fact, throughout the Western world, we have an economy-led agricultural system that produces very much more than we can eat, and then keeps the price of what we *do* eat artificially high and destroys the rest. Intensive farming practice has also robbed countless thousands of acres of agricultural land of its natural fertility, leaving farmers dependent on chemicals that pollute and damage the environment, consumers and themselves. The result is that the true cost of food to each individual is actually even higher than the falsely inflated price paid at the check-out. One way or another, we all meet the cost of dealing with the pollution, cleaning up the environment, repairing the roads and treating the bodies made ill by a diet rich in fat, sugar, additives and food-industry profit.

It is obvious to anyone who has observed nature that, if you take out more than you need from any natural system, you will ultimately harm yourself. It is also obvious that nature favours local eating of locally produced foods.

This book therefore recommends the eating of organic produce whenever possible. Not just because it tastes better; not just because it is more nutritious[2]; not just because it is free of potentially harmful chemical residues; but because organic farming makes plain common sense. Instead of taking goodness out of the soil and putting potentially harmful chemicals into people, it puts goodness back in the soil and takes potentially harmful chemicals out of our diet. Instead of paying for unripe or artificially treated produce to be transported halfway around the world, it pays local farmers to produce fresh, ripe produce for local consumers. Instead of hiding its true costs in direct and indirect taxation, its price includes the added bonus of healthier soil, a healthier environment and a healthier body.

Unfortunately, though widespread use of organic food production methods would improve life for farmers, consumers and nature (and would put an end to the institutionalized destruction of good food that is part of the current system), it would have a considerable impact on those food producers who believe that pendulums only swing one way. We have, therefore, to accept that the current balance of forces tends to favour the status quo, which means that organic produce remains an apparently expensive, hard to obtain luxury for most of us.

Despite this, there is still a lot that we, as individuals, can do to improve the quality of our diet and to hasten the development of a more rational, humane and sustainable food production system. We can:

1. Always choose fresh produce (organic or not) unless there really is no alternative to a processed product.

2. Go out of our way to find sources of truly local produce in our area (markets, smallholders, farm shops, roadside stalls, pick-your-own, friends, neighbours, relations, etc.)

---

[2]Weight for weight, organic produce tends to contain less water than non-organic and therefore provides a more concentrated source of essential nutrients.

3. Never buy an imported version of food that could be produced locally or nationally, seeking out home-grown produce whenever possible.

4. Always eat plenty of what is in season, avoiding costly out-of-season imports whenever possible.

5. Find and support local organic growers to the maximum extent of our budget. Some organic farmers operate a 'box' system where a selection of the week's produce is chosen and packed – and perhaps even delivered – by the farmer at a fixed weekly cost.

6. Find out about local barter networks (LETS schemes[3]) in our area and investigate local allotments and other community-based 'grow your own' possibilities.

Remember, the important thing about organic food is not what's in it, it's what's *not* in it. It tastes better, provides a more concentrated source of nutrients and comes from an agricultural system that is sustainable. If we all started buying it, it would even be cheap...

6. *Is there such a thing as first and second class proteins?*

There is a popular myth in Western society that the protein in milk, eggs and meat is of a higher quality than that in plants. Some people still think that only protein derived from animal products should be described as first class. These ideas are wrong and based on out-dated science. Research has shown clearly that plant foods are entirely adequate as sole sources of protein in the human diet and have the added advantage of being low in saturated fat and salt and high in fibre and other important nutrients. *All* grains, legumes[4], vegetables, fruits, nuts and seeds contain *all* the essential amino acids necessary for human health. Millions of people on the planet use only wheat, rice, corn or potatoes as their main protein sources and live healthy lives. Horses, elephants, bison, moose, gorillas and many other long-lived, well-muscled creatures build their remarkable physiques on a diet consisting wholly of plant foods.

As long as you eat a sufficient *amount* of plant food to meet your daily calorie needs, you are bound to eat more than enough protein. The average

[3]LETS (Local Exchange Trading System) is an international barter movement, particularly active in Canada, Australia and the UK. Started in 1983 by a Canadian called Michael Linton, it now has thousands of participants worldwide.
[4]Peas and beans.

protein content in pulses (expressed as a percentage of total calories) is twenty-seven percent, in nuts and seeds thirteen percent, and in grains twelve percent. Since the World Health Organization recommend a daily protein intake of ten percent of daily calories, it is easy to see that plant foods can provide all the protein necessary for health. Nearly all plant foods, except for some fruits, contain more than ten percent of their calories in the form of protein (see Appendix One, page 191).

Gram for gram, soya flour contains more protein than beef steak; yeast extract contains more protein than cheese; peanuts contain more protein than bacon; lentils contain more protein than roast chicken; chick-peas contain more protein than duck; butterbeans contain more protein than plaice; muesli contains more protein than eggs; parsley contains more protein than cow's milk; spinach contains more protein than yoghurt (based on UK Ministry of Agriculture, Fisheries and Food figures).

In fact, plant protein is the primary protein source on the planet. Amino acids and proteins exist because bacteria in the soil take nitrogen from the air and convert it into a form which plants can use. By combining this nitrogen with hydrogen, oxygen, carbon (and perhaps some sulphur), plants produce amino acids. They then join up the amino acids into chemical chains, which we call protein. The rest of creation either eats this protein in its primary form as plant food, or gets it second-hand by eating animals who have built their bodies by eating the primary protein of plants. Even in the sea, plant life in the form of algae forms the first link in the food chain.

Primary (plant) protein is cheap to produce in large quantities. From any given suitable acreage, you can produce about twenty times as much plant protein as animal protein. One acre of land can grow 9,000 kg of potatoes. The same area growing cattle feed will produce only 75 kg of beef. By eating secondary protein recycled through animal bodies, we waste up to ninety percent of the original plant protein. What is more, we lose ninety-six percent of the original calories, one hundred percent of the original fibre and one hundred percent of the original carbohydrate. 7.5 kg of grain and soya beans, used as animal feed, only produces 0.5 kg of meat on the plate.

With water becoming an ever more precious resource, it is worth remembering that producing a day's worth of animal-based food for one human being uses over 15,000 L of water. To produce the nutritional equivalent with plant-based food requires only 1,150 L. In other words, it takes less water to produce a year's supply of plant protein than it does to produce a one-month supply of animal protein.

Given the facts, it is important that the myth of the first class protein is laid to rest, and the best way to do this is to look at how it came about.

In the late 1800s, when the new science of organic chemistry was all the rage, scientists discovered how to extract protein from foodstuffs. As time went on, they were able to analyse the amino-acid composition of food proteins and make comparisons between these and the proteins found in human tissues. Having discovered that the combinations of amino acids in milk, eggs and meat were very similar to those found in human tissues, they made an understandable but wrong assumption – that this similarity made milk, eggs and meat the most suitable proteins for human diets.

These ideas were supported by experiments on rats in the 1930s, which appeared to show that plant proteins were 'deficient' in certain amino acids. Baby rats fed only on plant proteins had to be given amino acid supplements before they would grow properly. These observations led to the idea that plant proteins were somehow 'incomplete' and of lower 'biological value' than animal proteins, causing nutritional scientists to regard milk, eggs and meat as the protein 'benchmarks' by which all other proteins should be judged.

This research was deeply flawed, however, because it failed to take account of the simple fact that baby rats grow forty times faster than baby humans, and therefore require much more highly concentrated protein in their food. Rat's milk contains up to forty-nine percent of its calories in the form of protein, so plant food (containing between ten and thirty percent of protein calories) could never have supported baby rat growth without amino acid supplementation.

The fact that more highly concentrated animal-derived proteins could support the growth of weanling rats tells us nothing about the suitability of animal-derived foods as protein sources for human diets. Human breast milk contains only five to eight percent of its calories in the form of protein, so if we applied the logic of these early experiments we would have to conclude that human breast milk does not provide enough protein for human infants!

As already mentioned, it is now known that humans need just ten percent or less of their calorie intake to be in the form of protein. It is also known that, in order to grow and be healthy, we need to eat proteins containing different proportions of amino acids to those found in our own body tissues. What the early researchers did not understand was that the differences in amino acid composition between animal-based and plant-based foods did not mean that plant foods were of a lower nutritional quality. As long as calorie needs are met, it is easy for human beings to get ample protein from nearly all plant foods. All plants contain all necessary amino acids, even if individual amounts vary from plant to plant.

This means that not only is it unnecessary to supplement plant-based diets with animal-derived produce to ensure adequate protein intake, but there is also no truth in the idea that plant protein sources have to be combined in meals to make them 'complete'. (In normal circumstances, our bodies are able to make most of the amino acids we need for health, but eight – the so-called *essential amino acids* – have to be obtained from food. Essential amino acids are found in all plant and animal-based foods but, gram for gram, cereals, nuts and seeds contain less of the essential amino acid lysine than animal protein, although they are high in the essential amino acid, methionine. Pulses are rich in lysine and relatively low in methionine. The theory was that combining pulses with cereals, nuts or seeds at each meal would make the total protein eaten more 'complete'.)

Whilst 'protein combining' may reduce the overall *amount* of protein containing food that we need to eat to keep the body in positive protein balance, experiments on humans show clearly that even diets based on single plant sources of protein (eg. rice) will supply an adult with enough of all the essential amino acids. According to leading sources, including the American Dietetic Association, it is not necessary to combine protein foods at each meal because amino acids obtained from food can combine with amino acids made in the body to fulfil our needs over time.

The originator of the idea of protein combining, Frances Moore Lappé, never intended her work to convey the impression that animal-derived protein was superior to plant protein. In the tenth edition of her book, *Diet for a Small Planet*[5] she said:

> In combating the myth that meat is the only way to get high quality protein, I reinforced another myth. I gave the impression that in order to get enough protein without meat, considerable care was needed in choosing foods. Actually, it is much easier than I thought.

However, Western government food and agriculture policies – increasingly geared towards the rearing of animals to provide protein since the end of the Second World War – make it hard for most people to shake off old protein prejudices. Dietary research is still carried out on the basis that milk and eggs are 'standard' proteins – because they are similar in composition to human proteins – despite the widely acknowledged fact that human body protein composition does not reflect human dietary protein needs.

Because plant-based foods are less concentrated sources of protein than animal-based foods, and because the presence of fibre and other substances in plant foods may slightly reduce the amount of protein absorbed by the body from a plant-protein meal, the enormous benefits of eating plant protein are ignored by many people who remain convinced that 'more is

[5]Ballantine Books, 1981.

better'. Since plant protein always comes naturally packaged with other important nutrients, it is actually an advantage that you need to eat more plant-based foods than animal-based foods to meet your protein needs. By eating more vegetables, grains, pulses and fruits, you can be sure of eating all the other things that are good for your health *as well as* protein, ie. complex carbohydrates, essential fatty acids, fibre, vitamins, minerals and trace elements. You will also avoid eating high levels of cholesterol and saturated fat.

Even though animal proteins are still being heavily advertised, an increasing number of people are beginning to doubt their value. The uncertainty surrounding growth hormones for cattle, and Bovine Spongiform Encephalopathy (BSE), is making people consume less red meat. Chicken is promoted as a healthy alternative to red meat, but it still contains much more saturated fat than vegetable protein sources; intensively-reared chickens in Europe and America are also often fed female hormones to increase their weight. In today's polluted world, even fish – a very concentrated protein source – may contain toxic chemicals known to cause cancer, kidney failure, nerve damage and birth defects. Disturbing numbers of fish have been shown to contain heavy metals (arsenic, methylmercury, aluminium, cadmium), hydrocarbons (PCBs, pesticides, herbicides, dioxin, etc.) and radioactive contaminants. Furthermore, it is common practice among fishermen to spray dying fish in the holds of their ships with antibiotics and 'farmed' fish may also be treated with dyes and antibiotics.

To summarize, the concept that plant protein is incomplete is a myth, as is the idea of plant protein being second class. The suggestion that plant protein is indigestible is a distraction. There is no such thing as a first or second class protein. Plant proteins may have a different composition from our own body proteins, but they are good for us *because* they are different.

Plants provide us with primary protein. They are the fundamental high-quality protein sources on the planet. Plants contain all the amino acids necessary for health. Eat enough plants to meet your calorie needs and you will certainly eat enough protein. To quote George Bernard Shaw, 'Think of the fierce energy concentrated in an acorn. You bury it in the ground, and it explodes into a giant oak. Bury a sheep, and nothing happens but decay!'

7. *How much protein do I need to eat to be healthy?*

The word 'protein' is derived from the Greek word meaning 'to be in first place' and, thanks to protein-driven government food and agriculture policies and strong advertising, many Westerners still believe that they must eat large amounts of protein each day to sustain life and strength.

Of course, we do all need to consume a certain amount of daily protein, and severe protein deficiency is rightly associated in our minds with the worst effects of starvation, conjuring up pictures of emaciated children with distended tummies; but it is really very rare in the West to see anyone actually protein-deficient. On the contrary, it is becoming apparent that too much protein in the diet may lead to health problems, and protein excess may be an important factor in the rising incidence of osteoporosis (see below) and other diseases of civilization in our society. World health statistics show that human high protein meat-eating populations do not, as a rule, live as long as vegetarian populations and research also suggests an association between red meat consumption and the risk of heart attack, stroke and bowel cancer.

Nevertheless, it is difficult to assess exactly how much protein any one individual needs on a daily basis. Protein is used in many ways by the body, and requirements vary greatly according to circumstances and eating habits.

The first attempt at defining a recommended protein intake for the UK population (just after the Second World War) was based on the rather odd assumption that, since no-one in the UK was actually suffering from protein deficiency, the average amount eaten by the population each day was the right amount. This approach was also adopted in America, with the result that American recommendations for daily protein intake were set (and remain today) considerably higher than the British.

It was also assumed (particularly in the United States) that if some protein is good for you, then lots must be great. This led to the inclusion of 'dietary safety margins' in recommended intake figures, a subject that still provokes controversy in the scientific community. One passionate and outspoken nutritional commentator, Dr David Reuben, when asked who it was that actually needed the high allowance of protein recommended in the USA, answered:

> The people who sell meat, fish, cheese, eggs, chicken, and all the other high prestige and expensive sources of protein. Raising the amount of protein you eat by 30% raises their income by 30%. It also increases the amount of protein in the sewers and septic tanks of your neighbourhood by 30% as you merrily urinate away everything that you can't use that very day. It also deprives the starving children of the world of the protein that would save their lives.

A number of other assumptions were also made, which still affect our thinking on this subject. For example, it was assumed that men need more protein than women and children because they engage in more muscular activity. In fact, it has since been shown that more muscular activity does not, in itself, require extra protein intake. In the average Western family, it is not the adult male who needs the most protein – it is the children and childbearing women, who use protein for growth and breast milk production (because proteins are nature's building blocks).

Research and debate over how much protein we should eat continues to this day, and dietary protein recommendations are constantly under review. Despite the efforts of the scientists concerned, it is still proving difficult to marry the conclusions of those who study the diets of populations with the calculations of those who study the intimate biology of protein metabolism.

The situation is further complicated by the fact that any widely agreed change in recommended protein intakes would have a considerable impact on the economics of farming and food supply. As things stand, the average meat-eating Briton consumes eight cows, thirty-six pigs, thirty-six sheep and five hundred and fifty poultry birds in an average lifetime, as well as fish and large amounts of protein-containing vegetables. The average meat-eating American eats twenty-one cows, twelve sheep, fourteen pigs, nine hundred chickens and 454 kg of assorted birds and sea creatures during their life, in addition to vegetable protein sources. So it is clear that any change (whether towards less overall protein consumption or towards less animal protein consumption) would have important effects on society and on the international economy.

There is now more or less general agreement that a diet containing ten percent of its calories in the form of protein is more than adequate for people of all ages and it is, in fact, very unusual to find societies in the West whose daily protein intakes do not exceed this level. However, from a world perspective, many millions of people lead healthy lives on diets containing five percent or less of their calories in the form of protein.

Nature would seem to provide evidence that high protein intakes are neither necessary nor desirable for human health. Human breast milk contains only between five and eight percent of its calories as protein, and this is obviously sufficient to sustain the growth needs of the human baby. Protein requirements decrease significantly after infancy, as the rate of growth slows down, so the true protein requirement for the human adult may be only four percent of daily calories (except for pregnant and lactating women). What is more, nature would seem to be suggesting that, though they are very valuable to us, 'high protein' foods are not really *meant* to be consumed frequently in large amounts. In nature, nuts have hard shells, grains need harvesting and milling, and animals need to be hunted, killed and prepared.

8. *Saturated fats, hydrogenated fats, trans fats, cholesterol, unsaturated fats, essential fatty acids – what are they and are they OK to eat?*

Human beings like fat. It gives a texture to food – especially sweet food – that many of us regard as sensuous and luxurious, and on average, we all eat about 100 grams of it a day in one form or another. In other words, fat provides over forty percent of the total food energy intake for many Westeners, and about one quarter of this comes from dairy products.

However, the general consensus amongst scientists, nutritionists, public health workers and clinicians of all sorts is that:

1. We eat *too much* fat – which increases our risk of suffering serious illness such as heart disease, cancer and diabetes;

2. Too much of the fat we eat is of a type that increases our risk of suffering serious disease.

Since fat-related disease is so common in 'developed' countries – for example, coronary heart disease *alone* causes twenty-seven percent of all deaths in England and Wales, accounts for ten percent of all working days lost due to illness, costs the United Kingdom £500 million in medical treatment per year and a further £250 million in sickness benefit – the level of fat consumption in Western society is a major health issue. Unfortunately, the huge volume of research material now available (and the many different roles that fats play within our bodies) makes it hard for most people to understand which fats are good for us and which are bad. Does too much cholesterol in the blood cause heart disease, or does too little put us at risk of cancer? Does fish oil prevent heart attacks, or does it raise our blood cholesterol levels and cause the production of 'free radicals'? What is the difference between all the different sorts of fat, and how much should we eat of which sort?

To help clear up the confusion, here is some jargon busting.

Fat The word fat can be used to describe a large variety of greasy substances that don't dissolve in water but, as far as diet is concerned, fat is used as a general term to describe edible fatty substances that are solid at room temperature; these include butter, margarine, lard and the fatty parts of meat. In chemical terms, edible fats are made up of chemicals called triacylglycerols, but the human body also contains many other sorts of fat, which it makes out of the raw materials obtained from food. Fats are used by the body in many different ways. They are a ready store of energy, form important components of our body tissues and provide the basis for the manufacture of many important chemicals and hormones. Fat in our diet also makes it possible for us to absorb and use vitamins A, D, E and K (the fat soluble vitamins) from our food.

Oil Oils are edible fats that are *liquid* at room temperature, eg. olive oil, sunflower oil and grapeseed oil. Like the solid edible fats, they are also made up of triacylglycerols, and the only difference between edible fats and edible oils is in the types of fatty acid from which they are made. As we explain below, solid fats contain more saturated fatty acids whilst oils contain more unsaturated fatty acids[6].

Invisible fats Not all fat in our diet is 'visible' to us. Biscuits, cakes, mayonnaise, sausages, potato crisps and many other processed foods have fat (often a lot of fat) incorporated into them during their cooking or manufacture, but this fat is not usually obvious to us from the outside.

Fatty acids The edible fats and oils in our diet are made of chemicals called triacylglycerols. These are in turn made up of smaller molecules called fatty acids. Fatty acids consist of a chain of carbon atoms with some hydrogen and oxygen atoms attached in various places. About sixteen different types of fatty acid are found in the various triacylglycerols that make up our dietary fats and oils.

Saturated fatty acids A saturated fatty acid is a fatty acid that contains the maximum possible number of hydrogen atoms. The more saturated fatty acids a fat contains, the more likely it is to be solid at room temperature. Animal fats (including butter, lard and suet) contain high amounts of saturated fatty acids, as do solid vegetable fats like coconut oil. Since they can be made in the body, saturated fatty acids are not necessary in the human diet.

Unsaturated fatty acids An unsaturated fatty acid is a fatty acid in which two or more hydrogen atoms have been removed and replaced by what chemists call 'double bonds'. The name 'double bond' refers to a particular way of joining together links in a chemical chain.

Fatty acids with one double bond in their carbon chain are called mono-unsaturated fatty acids (MUFAs) and these are found in varying proportions in many animal, fish and vegetable fats. Oils rich in MUFAs (eg. olive oil) are usually thick liquids at room temperature. Like saturated fatty acids, MUFAs can be made in the body, so they are not a necessary component of the human diet.

Fatty acids with two or more double bonds in their carbon chains are

---

[6]The oil used in car engines is made up of different sorts of chemicals called hydrocarbons.

called polyunsaturated fatty acids (PUFAs). Plants provide the richest sources of PUFAs in the human diet, and oils rich in PUFAs – plant oils such as sunflower, corn, safflower and soya bean – are always liquid at room temperature. The proper functioning of our body cells depends on PUFAs and because of this, most of our tissues contain chemicals (enzymes) which convert saturated fatty acids into polyunsaturates. Table FA1 below shows the proportions of saturated fatty acids, mono-unsaturated fatty acids and polyunsaturated fatty acids in some common foods.

Table FA1 Fatty acid composition of some fats and oils

	Fatty acids (grams per 100g food)		
	SFA	MUFA	PUFA
Vegetable			
Coconut	85.2	6.6	1.7
Cottonseed	25.6	21.3	48.1
Maize, corn	16.4	29.3	49.3
Olive	14.0	69.7	11.2
Palm	45.3	41.6	8.3
Peanut	18.8	47.9	28.5
Rapeseed	5.4	64.3	24.8
Safflower seed	10.2	12.6	72.1
Soyabean	14.1	24.3	56.7
Sunflower seed	13.1	31.8	50.0
Wheatgerm oil	14.3	11.3	44.6
Pure vegetable margarines			
polyunsaturated	19.1	15.9	60.2
hard	28.8	37.9	9.8
soft	25.6	33.7	17.9
Animal			
Butter	49.0	26.1	2.2
Cooking fat	40.0	40.2	14.1
Dripping, beef	42.5	48.1	4.1
Lard	41.8	41.7	9.0
Low-fat spread	11.0	15.5	12.1
Margarine			
(mixed animal/vegetable oils)			
hard	29.8	34.6	13.8
soft	24.5	36.5	15.8
Suet	56.7	36.6	1.2

(UK Ministry of Agriculture, Fisheries and Food. The Composition of Foods)

ct>>>

YOU ARE WHAT YOU EAT

Essential Fatty Acids Two particular types of polyunsaturated fatty acid, linoleic and alpha-linolenic, cannot be made by the human body but are nevertheless vital to human health. Since we can only obtain them from food, they are called essential fatty acids (EFAs). EFAs are important components of all body cells (particularly brain cells) and are vital for the normal growth and development of the foetus during pregnancy and of the baby during infancy.

EFAs are also used by the body to produce a range of important chemicals called eicosanoids. Eicosanoids (such as the prostaglandins) form an essential part of the control mechanisms which make our blood clot when we bleed and which break down blood clots when they form obstructions in our blood vessels (thromboses). They are also vital to our capacity to react to injury and tissue damage. EFAs are found in abundance in vegetable oils (eg. sunflower oil, safflower oil, wheatgerm oil, soyabean oil and corn oil) and in green leaves, such as lettuce, cabbage and spring greens.

Hydrogenated and trans fats When making processed foods, food manufacturers often need to use solid or semi-solid fats in order to give the right textures and consistencies to their products and to ensure a good shelf-life. However, it is in the interests of all manufacturers to use low-cost raw materials. Many vegetable oils are cheap and in good supply, but are too liquid for most product applications; so manufacturers have developed ways of changing the physical properties of vegetable and other inexpensive oils to make them more suitable to their needs.

Because saturated fats tend to be solid at room temperature, one way of producing a more solid fat from a low-cost polyunsaturated oil is to mix some saturated fat with it. Since animal fats are high in saturates, and since cheap vegetable oils are readily available, the words, 'contains animal and vegetable fat' are seen on the labels of many processed foods (cakes, biscuits, margarines, etc.).

A second way of making a polyunsaturated oil more solid is to make it more saturated by adding hydrogen to it – in other words, by hydrogenating it. Hydrogenated and partially hydrogenated fats are ingredients of many processed foods and can be produced by a variety of industrial methods. The chemical and physical manipulations involved in hydrogenation cause other changes to the fat, however. Some of the double bonds in the fatty acid chains are altered in shape and turn into what are known as trans double bonds. Trans fats (ie. fats containing trans double bonds) in food are now generally considered to be bad for health even though, from the manufacturer's point of view, they enhance the effects of hydrogenation

82

because trans fats also tend to be solid at room temperature, like saturated fats[7].

A third way to alter the physical characteristics of a polyunsaturated oil to make it a more suitable processed food ingredient is to use emulsifiers. An emulsion is a smooth mixture of oil and water (like salad dressing after it has been well mixed) and emulsifiers are substances that stop the oil and water separating in emulsions. Many modern margarines 'high in polyunsaturates' achieve their buttery consistency because of the use of modern emulsifier technology, which avoids the need for hydrogenation.

Cholesterol Cholesterol has acquired an odd reputation in the last part of the twentieth century. In the body, it is an essential constituent of cell membranes, and is also a raw material necessary for the production of bile and various hormones. Chemically, it is a sort of hybrid between alcohol and fat, and it is only found in animal tissues. Plants contain no cholesterol. Because it performs multiple roles in the body, cholesterol is continually being transported from one place to another in the blood, carried on the back of chemicals called lipoproteins. Our body makes all the cholesterol it needs without us having to eat any in our diet.

If we eat a low-fat diet, relatively rich in polyunsaturated fats (from vegetables and plant oils), cholesterol accumulates in the cell membranes of our nerves and other tissues – in other words, where it is supposed to be. However, if we eat a high-fat diet, rich in saturated fat (ie. containing animal and dairy products), the amount of cholesterol being transported in our bloodstream is increased and we become prone to atheroma and thrombosis, which block our blood vessels and can produce angina and heart attacks.

Eating a lot of cholesterol in our diet does not, in itself, significantly increase our risk of heart disease. What definitely does increase this risk, is eating a lot of the *sort* of foods that contain high levels of cholesterol – animal-based foods – since it is these foods that are high in fat *overall* and particularly high in saturated fat. The idea that a low blood cholesterol may be a cancer risk has been shown to be false. A recently reported study of British men, followed up over fifteen years, showed that the deaths in patients with low cholesterol were due to other causes, including poor lifestyle associated with smoking and heavy drinking.

---

[7]One of the reasons why beef and dairy products contain so much saturated fat is that most of the polyunsaturated fat that cows eat is hydrogenated – made more saturated – by bacteria that live in their stomachs. This bacterial hydrogenation also produces a lot of trans double bonds, so cows end up absorbing large amounts of hydrogenated and trans fats into their bodies, which are passed on to us in meat and milk products.

Fish Oils Lean fish (plaice, sole, cod, etc.) tend to store their body fat in their livers. Oily fish (eg. mackerel, herring and salmon) store their fat in their flesh. Since fish liver is not a common food (cod-liver oil having mercifully gone out of fashion), the best way to eat fish oil is to eat oily fish. The oils contained in all fish (lean or oily) are very high in polyunsaturated fatty acids, particularly of a type called 'omega three fatty acids'.

Although it has taken several pages to describe the different sorts of fat in our diet, when it comes to eating them, it only takes one sentence to sum up the best evidence: **Eat less saturated fat, avoid hydrogenated and trans fats and include some polyunsaturated oils in your diet.** In practical terms, for most of us this means:

1. Reducing the intake of meat, milk, cheese and eggs – the main sources of saturated fat in the Western diet.

2. Avoiding (or at least reducing the intake of) butter, which is high in saturated fat and which – contrary to the impression sometimes given – contains about five percent trans fats. (The fact that some margarines are still made from a blend of animal fats, hydrogenated oils and non-hydrogenated oils – and thus contain high levels of trans fats – has been taken by some to imply that butter is healthier than margarine. In fact, both butter and the old type of margarine are not good for health; butter is naturally high in saturated fats and naturally contains trans fats. The solution is to use only spreads made from non-hydrogenated oils that are high in polyunsaturates.)

3. Avoiding margarines that contain hydrogenated oils and trans fats. (There are now several brands available that contain no hydrogenated oils and are free – or virtually free – of trans fats. This information is usually clearly advertised on the packet.)

4. Avoiding (as far as possible) processed foods which contain animal fats or hydrogenated vegetable oils.

5. Eating a diet which contains some sunflower or safflower oil and plenty of green, leafy vegetables, to ensure a good supply of essential fatty acids.

If you follow this advice, you will automatically reduce the level of cholesterol in your blood, particularly the type known as LDL cholesterol, which is strongly linked with heart disease. This cholesterol-lowering effect can be further enhanced by avoiding refined carbohydrates and sugar, and eating more complex carbohydrates and soluble fibre in the form of vegetables and fruits.

These guidelines will also help you to reduce the total amount of fat that you eat. In this way, you not only decrease your risk of coronary heart disease, you also reduce your chances of developing cancer. Saturated fat – particularly animal fat – has been shown to increase the risk of bowel cancer, kidney cancer, ovarian cancer and cancer of the uterus. Eating less fat overall also helps in avoiding obesity and conditions associated with obesity, such as late-onset diabetes.

Finally, a few more words about fish oils. The observation that Eskimos eating a traditional Eskimo diet, high in fat, but rich in oily fish, seem to be at less risk than the average Westerner of dying of coronary heart disease, has given rise to the suggestion that some of the fatty acids in fish oil – long chain n-3 fatty acids, such as eicosapentaenoic acid (EPA) and docosahexaenoic acid – may make fish oil protective against coronary thrombosis. This, in turn, has led to the enthusiastic recommendation of oily fish or fish oil supplements by some nutritional commentators and nutritional supplement companies. We do not share this enthusiasm for the following reasons.

1. Although Eskimos eat a lot of fat in their diet, their total intake of saturated fat is about fifty percent less than that of the average Westerner (fat from oily fish is highly polyunsaturated). Increasing fish oil intake without also reducing saturated fat intake is unlikely to have any significant effect on the development of coronary heart disease.

2. Taking fish oil does not reduce blood cholesterol levels. Indeed, taking 6 grams or more a day of fish oil supplements can actually increase blood cholesterol.

3. The effect of fish oils on cardiac death seems to be more to do with a reduction in the chances of dying from the complications of a heart attack than with a reduction in the chances of having a heart attack in the first place.

4. Though the long chain, n-3 fatty acids in fish oil certainly do reduce the tendency of the blood to clot and cause thrombosis, so do other polyunsaturated fatty acids, such as linoleic and alpha linolenic acids (found in vegetable oils and green leaves respectively). Alpha-linolenic acid can even be converted to fish oil type EPA in the body.

5. Taking fish oils in a concentrated form may cause excessive production of free radicals (see question 9 overleaf), which can cause degeneration of tissues, if present in large quantities over a long period of time. Unlike fish oils, plant sources of polyunsaturated fatty acids are high in natural anti-oxidants, which combat the effects of free radicals.

9. *Should I be taking anti-oxidant supplements to protect against free radicals?*

Metabolism releases the energy contained in food to make our hearts beat, our muscles contract, our nerves conduct electricity and our glands secrete hormones and other chemicals. In the process we use up oxygen breathed in from the air and produce water and carbon dioxide as waste products. Put simply:

$$Food + Air = Work + Waste Products$$

Some of the chemical reactions involved in metabolism also generate by-products known as free radicals. Free radicals are molecules carrying an unbalanced electrical charge, and they have a strong tendency to react with any nearby chemical that offers the chance of greater electrical stability.

The membranes that form the walls of all our body cells contain poly-unsaturated fatty acids, which are particularly prone to react with free radicals in a chemical reaction known as oxidation. Since fatty acid oxidation by free radicals can cause severe damage, our cell membranes also contain built-in safety devices called *anti*-oxidants, which mop up any free radicals produced during metabolism before they can do any harm. One of the body's most important anti-oxidants – vitamin E – is found in large amounts in all cell membranes. Vitamin A (in its plant 'carotenoid' form), vitamin C, and a selenium containing chemical called glutathione peroxidase, also have important anti-oxidant actions.

The current interest in the link between anti-oxidants and health – and in the link between free radicals and disease – has been stimulated by research, which suggests that vitamin E may be able to slow the progress of Parkinson's disease, reduce the severity of some neurological disorders, slow down the progress of cataracts, improve mobility in arthritis and reduce tissue damage during surgery. There is also some evidence that anti-oxidants (including vitamin E) play an important role in preventing coronary heart disease and cancer. What is more, chemicals containing free radicals are common contributors to late twentieth century air pollution; cigarette smoke alone contains huge amounts. So there is clearly a case for making sure we get plenty of anti-oxidants in our diet, even though the nature of free radical/anti-oxidant reactions is not yet fully understood.

Vegetables, fruits, nuts, seeds and cold pressed oils, such as safflower and olive oil are the best natural sources of anti-oxidants, including vitamin A, vitamin C, vitamin E and selenium. If you base your diet on the ten Personal Eating Principles, you will ensure a rich daily supply of anti-oxidants without the need to invest in dietary supplements.

10. *Is raw food better for health than cooked food?*

In today's pre-packed society, many people find the idea of a raw food diet attractive. Since humankind sustained itself through evolution by 'eating wild', some say that we should return to taking our food 'as it comes', as an antidote to modern civilization and its diseases of excess and plenty. Raw food diets have certainly become popular in the management of various diseases, including arthritis, cancer and diabetes, and even people not particularly interested in health and diet value their daily helping of crisp, raw salad or fresh fruit.

However, the concept of raw food being good for you is relatively modern. Just one hundred years ago, the word 'salad' referred to cooked greens and, for centuries before our era, cooking was regarded as the cornerstone of good food hygiene. Since cooking reduces the bulk of food, making it easier to chew and (to some extent) digest, it has made it possible for 'civilised' man to spend much less time eating than would be necessary on an exclusively raw food diet. The cooking fire or the kitchen are also at the heart of many communities – places of warmth and companionship.

From the point of view of naturopathic nutrition, there are three good reasons for increasing the amount of raw food in our diet, where possible.

1. Nature provides raw food and every other species on the planet survives very well on it. Following nature's example in this respect would undoubtedly suggest that our food is meant to be eaten raw.

2. Cooked food is dead food. Heating destroys the living cells that make up plant and animal tissues. Whilst there is no scientific evidence to suggest that this makes any difference, we all recognize the special quality of really fresh foods like raw carrot, crisp lettuce, fresh cucumber and crunchy celery. From the naturopathic point of view, this quality is vitality. The fact that our senses tell us that vital food is good for us suggests that we should try our best to eat it, whenever we have the choice.

87

3. Cooking alters the chemical nature of food and depletes it of various essential nutrients. The 'browning' of protein-containing food changes its protein structure and decreases the availability of certain amino acids (particularly the essential amino acid, lysine). Vitamins and minerals are lost into cooking water and some vitamins – for example C, thiamin and folic acid – are destroyed by heating. High temperature frying de-natures vitamin A and vitamin E, both of which are important anti-oxidants. Although cooking makes the starches in plant foods more digestible (by making starch granules swell up and burst cell walls), when starchy foods are cooled, a part of the starch actually becomes less digestible, and has to spend more time in the bowel being broken down by microorganisms. Overheating or repeated heating of fats and oils turns them rancid and toxic.

Nevertheless, a diet consisting totally or mostly of raw food is not a practical proposition for many people these days, so it is important to know how to minimize any damaging effects that cooking might have on the nutritional qualities of our food.

As far as fresh ingredients are concerned (processed food products should always be prepared in accordance with the manufacturer's recommendations), the basic rule is to cook them as lightly as possible. Vitamin losses from vegetables can be minimized by putting them in water that is already boiling (instead of pre-soaking them or starting cooking in cold water). Vegetables and rice should be pre-washed as little as possible, consistent with good hygiene. Cooking vegetables in covered pans with minimal added water – after first briefly shallow-frying them in a little spiced oil – is also a good way of retaining their nutritional value (Indian cuisine being a marvellous example of maximum nutritional quality with minimal use of resources).

11. *How do I avoid suffering from wind?*

The gas responsible for flatulence and wind is produced by the fermentation of carbohydrates and proteins that have not been completely digested on their way through the gut. This fermentation is caused by microorganisms that live in our colons which, like microorganisms elsewhere in nature, have the job of clearing up left-over waste material from the environment. If they have to deal with large amounts of undigested materials, they produce large amounts of gas which can cause abdominal distension and discomfort.

If you suffer from excess wind, the answer is: a) cut down on food that contains sugars and starches that are not so easily digestible; b) avoid excessive protein intake; and c) prepare high-protein foods in such a way as to make them more readily digestible.

The following foods contain sugars and starches that may not be fully digested and so produce wind:

Milk	Chicory
Beans	Salsify
Peas	Unripe banana
Onions	Undercooked potato
Leeks	Undercooked sweetcorn
Artichokes	Unmilled seeds

Wholemeal bread is also more prone to cause wind than white bread. Of the high-protein foods, meats cause less wind when minced, and pulses cause less wind when properly soaked and cooked.

This information should not put you off the foods mentioned. Many people can eat all of them without being troubled by flatulence. Some people find that cutting down on just one or two of the foods mentioned will solve their problem. So if you suffer from wind, we suggest that you experiment, cutting out some of the potentially less digestible foods from your diet for a couple of weeks, seeing if things improve and then eating them again to see if things get worse.

12. *If I choose not to eat any animal produce, won't I get deficient in some important vitamins?*

Not if you follow the diet recommendations set out in the previous chapter.

The debate about animal-produce-free diets and nutrient deficiency involves just two vitamins: vitamin D and vitamin B12.

Vitamin D is necessary to help us absorb calcium from our food, and a deficiency can lead to softening of the bones and deformity (known as rickets in children and osteomalacia in adults). Although vitamin D is added to a number of fortified foods (such as margarines and breakfast cereals), only a few foods (eg. eggs, butter and oily fish) contain vitamin D naturally. However, vitamin D in food is not necessary for most people (even babies), since we all produce vitamin D internally by the action of sunlight on our skin. Even 'skyshine' on a cloudy day causes vitamin D production. So, whether or not we choose to eat animal produce, the best way to ensure adequate vitamin D is to spend some time each day in the open air. Black people and Asian vegetarians living in countries where climate restricts exposure to daylight seem to be slightly more at risk of vitamin D deficiency than Caucasians, and there is also some evidence that babies, after four to six months of age, fed on breast milk alone may need some extra vitamin D to ensure proper nourishment. However, there is no evidence that an animal-produce free diet in itself increases the risk of vitamin D deficiency, as long as it provides sufficient calories and an adequate amount of protein – and as long as there is regular exposure to daylight. Fortified foods (margarines, plant milks, etc.) containing added non-animal vitamin D2 (ergocalciferol) can, of course, be used as extra insurance, where necessary.

The human dietary requirement for vitamin B12 has been the subject of debate for many years. The vitamin is used by cells that normally divide rapidly, such as those in the bone marrow, which produce our blood cells, and also by the cells that maintain the integrity of our nerve tissue. B12 deficiency may therefore cause anaemia and can, over a long period of time, also result in damage to the nervous system, particularly the spinal cord.

However, vitamin B12 deficiency caused by not eating enough is very rare indeed. Even people regularly eating just a quarter of the 'recommended' daily average amount seem to remain perfectly healthy. What is more, since we store vitamin B12 in our livers, most of us could live perfectly healthily on our liver B12 reserves for up to six years without eating any B12 at all (and we also have efficient mechanisms for conserving as much B12 as possible within our bodies).

The only relatively common cause of B12 deficiency is an inability to absorb it from the diet because of disease. Since B12 can't be absorbed from food without the presence of a chemical called intrinsic factor (which is produced by the stomach), and since the actual *process* of absorption takes place in the small intestine, damage to the stomach or to the small intestine (from disease or even surgery) may make it impossible to absorb B12. People unable to produce sufficient intrinsic factor in the first place also develop B12 deficiency, resulting in the condition known as pernicious anaemia.

It is a common misconception that vitamin B12 can only be obtained from animal foods. However, those animals that people 'rely' on to provide B12 are themselves pure vegetarians who must be getting *their* B12 from a *non*-animal food source. In fact, vitamin B12 is produced by microorganisms that live in the soil. Since grazing animals don't wash the grass they eat, they inevitably eat B12 producing organisms, which then take up residence within their digestive tracts. The B12 produced is absorbed and therefore appears in meat, milk and offal.

If we ate raw food (cooking reduces B12 content) straight from the wild or the soil without much cleaning or preparation – and if we weren't repeatedly exposed to antibiotics which kill many of the helpful bacteria that would otherwise inhabit our gut – we would also get our B12 quota from bacteria living in our small intestine. Even in today's sanitized society, there is evidence that people consuming a plant-food only diet consisting of organic, lightly washed produce are still able to obtain their B12 in this way.

However, since this way of eating is not available to most of us, it is important to know about other reliable B12 sources if we eat no meat, dairy products or fish. Recent research into the B12 content of various plant foods showed that edible seaweeds, fermented soya products and spirulina preparations, previously thought to be good non-animal sources of B12, actually contain little or no biologically active vitamin B12. The best advice for most one hundred percent vegetarians is, therefore, to make sure their diet contains some foods that are *fortified* with B12, such as certain yeast extracts, margarines, plant milks, soya products and breakfast cereals. This advice is particularly important for pregnant and breast-feeding women, and for babies who have been weaned, since vitamin B12 plays a vital role in normal growth and development[8]. However, it is not necessary to eat a product containing B12 every day; about three times a week is probably enough. It is also wasteful to take large amounts of vitamin B12 in the form of vitamin pills, since three micro-grams (millionths of a gram) is the most that anyone can absorb from any given meal.

Note: Folic acid, a B-group vitamin found in high concentrations in all plant-based diets, actually protects against the anaemia of vitamin B12 deficiency. The concern over B12 deficiency amongst adult vegans therefore relates only to the possibility of developing neurological problems over a long period of time, and to the healthy growth and development of their children.

13. *Should I be taking calcium supplements to avoid osteoporosis?*

Few topics in nutrition cause more argument amongst professionals than the role of calcium supplements in the prevention and treatment of osteoporosis. The lack of clear evidence one way or another often reduces the debate to a pantomime-like 'oh yes they do' – 'oh no they don't' level, and can leave the consumer vulnerable to incomplete or one-sided advice which

---

[8]There are also fortified non-animal derived infant feeding formulas available for times when breast feeding is not possible.

encourages considerable expenditure with little or no chance of real benefit. What is more, the narrowness of the discussion discourages people from taking effective preventive and remedial action for themselves, since many now believe that calcium supplements, pills and hormone replacement therapy are the only available anti-osteoporosis strategies.

There is no doubt that a good intake of calcium from the diet is important, and following the advice in the previous chapter will certainly ensure that you eat plenty. However, it is important to be aware of other aspects of the osteoporosis debate that are mentioned less often in the public discussion.

Osteoporosis is a condition in which the total amount of bone in the skeleton decreases, even though the bone that is left is normal in its composition. It leads to disabling fractures of the spine, hip and wrist and is particularly common in post-menopausal women in Western society. Despite what is commonly supposed, it is virtually impossible to produce osteoporosis by restricting calcium intake in the diet. It is also not possible to reduce post-menopausal bone loss simply by eating more calcium. So anyone wanting to reduce their risk of suffering the effects of osteoporosis needs to look beyond eating chalk and drinking milk for an effective answer.

1. It is important to realize that *using* the skeleton by keeping mobile and active is widely acknowledged to be one of the best insurances against bone loss and osteoporosis. It is common sense that anything not being used risks falling into decay and disrepair.

2. You should be aware that smoking and drinking are clearly related to an increased risk of developing osteoporosis.

3. There is a clear link between the consumption of too much protein – particularly animal protein – and the chances of developing osteoporosis. Osteoporosis is most common in precisely those countries with the highest protein intakes – the USA, the UK, Finland, Sweden and Denmark. It is also rampant amongst Eskimos, who survive largely on protein foods. Conversely, communities with low-protein diets – such as the Bantu in South Africa – have a very low incidence of osteoporosis even though their diet is also low in calcium.

The reason is that high protein intake causes loss of calcium in the urine, and the relationship between too much protein in the diet and loss of bone density is direct and consistent. Even with very high calcium intakes (eg. from supplements), excess protein in the diet is associated with a loss of calcium from the bones. In other words, the more protein you eat, the more calcium you will lose regardless of your calcium intake.

This is not to say that we should not eat protein. It simply means that we should not eat more than we need, and that we should be careful about the type of protein we consume. The higher levels of phosphorus and sulphur in meat increase calcium loss from the body; research comparing animal-protein-only diets with mixed and with vegetable-protein-only diets has shown that a higher intake of vegetable protein may protect against bone calcium loss and hence against osteoporosis[9]. This idea is supported by evidence that older Caucasian women who are vegetarians have a significantly higher total bone mass than meat eaters. Commenting on current research into osteoporosis, one of America's leading authorities on diet and disease, Dr John McDougass, has said:

'I would like to emphasize that the calcium-losing effect of protein on the human body is not an area of controversy in scientific circles. The many studies performed during the past fifty-five years consistently show that the most important dietary change that we can make if we want to create a positive calcium balance that will keep our bones solid is to decrease the amount of protein we eat each day. The important change is not to increase the amount of calcium we take in.'

To summarize, the best way to avoid osteoporosis is:

- To keep active;

- To cut down on (or, better, cut out) smoking and alcohol;

- To eat no more protein than you need each day (see question 7, page 76);

- To increase the proportion of vegetable to animal-derived protein in your diet.

There is no need to drink milk[10], eat cheese or take calcium supplements. Most plant foods contain calcium, and spinach, watercress, parsley, dried figs, nuts, seeds, molasses, seaweed and soya products are particularly good sources. Gram for gram, tofu contains four times more calcium than whole cow's milk, and the old idea that the extra fibre and phytate content in plant food may interfere significantly with calcium absorption is rejected by the

[9]Part of the protective effect of vegetables and fruits against osteoporosis may be due to the fact that vegetables and fruits contain boron, a chemical which tends to reduce urinary calcium loss and raise blood oestrogen levels.
[10]In any case, drinking too much cow's milk is a known risk factor for developing iron deficiency anaemia. Calcium in cow's milk interferes with the absorption of iron from the diet.

American Dietetic Association and UK authorities. Meat and fish contain only tiny amounts of calcium.

14. *Is soya safe?*

Reports casting doubt on the safety of different foods are common these days, and many people are confused about how seriously to take them. The trouble is that premature, incomplete, over-simplified or spin-doctored media accounts of highly technical nutritional research can make scientific possibilities look too much like scientific facts (much to the discomfort of scientists, who are usually very wary about linking effects with causes). The result is that more public attention is paid to what might be bad for us than what is known to be good for us.

In fact, since most people eat many different foods prepared in many different ways, the true effect of any single ingredient on any individual diet is very hard to assess. So it is probably wise to approach evidence about the safety of any particular food in much the same way as you would approach a strange dog; with respect but without fear. Most dogs turn out to be friendly, if treated sensibly…

The concern about soya relates to four scientific observations:

1. Raw soya beans contain phytates, which can affect the absorption of certain minerals from the diet.

2. Raw soya beans contain oestrogen-like substances.

3. Raw soya beans contain chemicals which decrease the efficiency of protein digestion.

4. Raw soya beans may contain relatively high levels of aluminium.

Let us look at each of these facts in turn.

1. Phytates are chemicals found in many different plant-based foods, but ninety percent of the phytates in the average diet come from cereal products, particularly those with a high bran content. The amount of phytate we consume can influence the amount of calcium, iron and zinc we absorb from food and this has given rise to the speculation that a diet containing too much phytate may lead to mineral deficiencies. Whilst this is a theoretical possibility, it is not what seems to happen in practice.

Many phytate-containing foods are rich in iron and, in the case of soya products, this counterbalances the inhibiting effect of phytates. What is more, vitamin C counteracts the effects of phytate on iron absorption, and a good diet always contains vitamin C. Also, phytates are not the only things that interfere with iron uptake: just one glass of milk can reduce iron absorption from a meal by half.

The American Dietetic Association and the Ministry of Agriculture, Fisheries and Foods in the UK have concluded that phytates in the diet are unlikely to have any detrimental effect on calcium levels in the body.

There is no evidence that people consuming varied, healthy diets high in phytates become zinc deficient. In fact, many high phytate foods – wholegrains, for example – contain high levels of zinc. An adequate protein intake provides added insurance against zinc deficiency by reducing the effects of phytate on zinc absorption.

2. Soya beans contain chemicals that are oestrogen 'lookalikes' and are thus a source of oestrogen-like chemicals in many diets. Chemicals that mimic oestrogens can be found in many plants, as well as in pesticides, detergents and some plastics. For adults, oestrogenic substances in food may well be a benefit to health, since there is evidence that they may protect against breast cancer and prostate cancer. On the other hand, they may decrease fertility to some extent, and the effects of phyto-oestrogens on babies that are fed on soya-milk formula foods are not known (although there are no reported cases of adverse effects).

3. Soya beans contain chemicals known as anti-trypsins, which can interfere with the digestion of protein in the small intestine. Sprouting, cooking or dehulling the beans destroys the anti-trypsins, so most available soya products are free from undesirable anti-trypsin effects on protein digestion.

4. Aluminium intake may be associated with an increased risk of developing Alzheimer's disease, which has given rise to concern over aluminium levels in the water supply, and over the long-term use of aluminium cookware. Soya beans contain some aluminium, with the amount depending on the type of soil in which they are grown. As a result, concentrated soya-based infant formula feeds contain significant – and possibly undesirable – amounts of aluminium.

On balance, for adults eating a varied diet – omnivore, lacto-ovo vegetarian or one hundred percent vegetarian – phytates, phyto-oestrogens, anti-trypsins and aluminium in soya products do not constitute a particular health risk. Soya beans are a useful and versatile source of protein and oil, and the preparation methods used to produce most soya-based foods minimize the possibility of undesirable side-effects.

However, with our current level of knowledge, it is probably advisable to regard soya-based infant formula foods with some caution, until more is known about the effects of phyto-oestrogens on the growing baby, and until the significance of their higher aluminium content is better understood.

15. *Can naturopathic nutrition help with weight loss?*

It is well-known that being overweight increases your chances of dying young, and slightly less well-known that being underweight also increases your chances of early death and disease. In the West, however, it is obesity that poses the major threat to health, and being overweight is clearly linked to heart disease, stroke, hypertension, late onset diabetes, gallstones, chest disease, osteo-arthritis and back problems.

However, before worrying about your weight, check whether you really do have anything to be concerned about. Here's a simple way of finding out (you may find it helpful to use a calculator).

1. Write down your weight in kilograms

2. Measure your height in metres (if you are 180 cm tall, your height in metres is 1.80), then multiply this number by itself.

3. Divide your weight in kilograms by your height in metres multiplied by itself, ie:

$$\frac{\text{Weight (in kilograms)}}{\text{Height} \times \text{Height (in metres)}}$$

The figure you come up with is known as your Body Mass Index.
Here is a worked example.

Your weight:	78 kilograms
Your height:	1.80 metres
Your height × itself	1.80 × 1.80 = 3.24
Your Body Mass Index	$\frac{78}{3.24} = 24.07$

If your Body Mass Index is between 20 and 25, your weight is fine; between 25 and 30, you are overweight; between 30 and 35, you are definitely obese; over 35, you are seriously overweight; and if less than 20, you are underweight.

If you find that you are overweight (or worse), deciding what to do about it is not always easy. There are hundreds (if not thousands) of books available on diet, dieting and weight loss (let alone countless magazine articles, weight loss supplements, slimming groups and clubs, etc.), but the fact that there are so many may suggest that no one is offering a complete and reliable weight-loss method that applies to everyone.

The reason for this is simple – whether we worry about our weight or not, most of us like eating what we like. If weight loss were approached in a completely scientific way (not taking account of preferences, prejudices, desires and personalities), losing weight would be no problem in most cases since it is a basic fact that if we regularly take in more food energy than we need, we gain weight and if we regularly take in less than we need, we lose weight. In scientific terms, therefore, slimming is a simple matter. If you want to lose weight, eat less and do more.

Applying this basic principle in real life is more complicated, however, and successful slimming methods (such as Weight Watchers) take account of the psychological aspects and practical difficulties involved. It may be very diffi-cult for someone whose dietary options are limited (by their work or domes-tic circumstances) to change what they eat; and it is certainly not advisable for a very obese person to take strenuous physical exercise, since this will merely cause exhaustion, without using up a significant amount of energy overall.

Nevertheless, there are a number of general principles which can be applied to any weight-loss regime to maximize the chances of success. These are:

1. *Take it slowly*: rapid weight loss can cause you to lose non-fatty tissue, as well as fat, and following a very restricted diet for long periods may deprive you of essential nutrients; 0.5 to 1 kilogram reduction in weight per week is ideal.

2. *Know what you are aiming for*: if you are overweight and can reduce your Body Mass Index to 25 (see page 96), that is enough. Super-thin does not necessarily mean super-healthy.

3. *Be realistic about how long it will take*: take your height in metres. Multiply this number by itself, then multiply the result by 25. This is your target weight in kilograms, if you are currently overweight.

Subtract your target weight from your current weight (in kilograms). The result is the *minimum* number of weeks that it should take you to reach your target weight. For example:

Your height: 1.75m
1.75m multiplied by itself: 3.06
3.06 × 25 = 76.5kg (your target weight).
Your current weight: 90kg
90 – 76.5 = 13.5

79.21

So in this example you should take at least thirteen and a half weeks to reach your target weight.

4. *When you weigh less, you need to eat less*: a stable weight is good for health, and research has shown that people whose weight remains more or less constant live longer than people whose weight is continually going up and down. If you do lose weight, it is important that your new, lower weight becomes your constant weight.

Recent evidence seems to suggest that dieting may alter brain chemistry in such a way as to distort our appetite control mechanisms, and these findings support the view that 'dieting makes you fat'. So to achieve stable weight loss requires two things: (1) a realization that a thinner body requires less calories each day than a fatter body; (2) an understanding that if you were overweight for any length of time before losing weight, your appetite will tell you that 'eating normally' is eating at least the amount that kept you overweight in the first place.

To maintain weight loss after dieting, therefore, you have to train your appetite to understand that eating a bit less is normal. This may take a few weeks, but the effort is amply rewarded by the physical, mental and emotional benefits that come from feeling more comfortable about your weight[11].

5. *Keep active*: the number of overweight people in the UK has doubled over the past ten years and recent research suggests that the modern tendency towards inactivity is just as important as too much food in causing obesity. Exercise – even walking or cycling – seems to have gone out of fashion, and the average person in Britain now sits and watches twenty-six hours of television a week, compared with just thirteen hours in the 1960s.

Without question, increased activity plays a vital role in the treatment and prevention of obesity. Whilst participating in sport and other forms of organized physical activity is regarded by many as the best way of taking exercise, a lack of sporting opportunity does not exclude the possibility of raising our daily activity level. Walking briskly whenever you can (eg. for short trips instead of taking the bus or the car), taking the stairs (up and down) instead

---

[11]To work out precisely how much less you should eat in calorie terms requires quite a complicated calculation. However, as a very rough guide, for every kilogram of weight loss, you need to reduce your daily calorie intake by about 20 kcals if you are a man, or 15 kcals if you are a woman, to maintain the lower weight. For example, if you are a woman who has reduced your weight from 80 kg to 60 kg, you will need to reduce your daily calorie intake by about 300 kcals a day (20 × 15) to remain stable at your new weight.

of lifts or escalators in shops, and doing some house and garden tasks manually instead of with machines can be more effective at using up calories than many forms of strenuous exercise.

Incidentally, some people worry that taking exercise will simply make them eat more. Whilst it is true that physical activity stimulates the appetite to some extent, the calories used up during non-strenuous exercise usually outnumber the extra calories eaten as a result by a considerable margin.

The Personal Eating Principles described in Chapter Seven are designed to help you maintain a constant, healthy weight. If you base your diet on these principles, you will be eating:

- Foods rich in essential nutrients, but low in fat-forming empty calories.

- A low-fat, high-fibre diet that satisfies your hunger without loading you with excess calories.

- A diet that is varied, affordable and full of vitality.

If you need to lose weight, you can apply the Personal Eating Principles to any reducing diet to ensure that you remain properly nourished whilst you are losing weight. Whichever method of losing weight you choose, you should also bear the following points in mind:

1. Long-term calorie controlled diets recommending an intake of less than 800 calories a day are too severe and may be harmful to health.

2. Reducing diets recommending an intake of more than 1500 calories per day are unlikely to be very effective.

3. If you can't be bothered with calorie counting, remember that for most people a reducing diet of 1000 to 1500 kcals per day is equivalent to cutting your current food consumption by between a third and a half. Using smaller plates, or serving yourself 'normally' and then removing between a third and a half of all the different foods on the plate (to be eaten later or recycled in other meals), are simple ways of cutting calories without all the fuss.

4. Most people find it better to keep to set meal and snack times, when dieting. Small and often is more healthy than starve and binge.

5. Weight loss can affect the action of some medicines. If you are taking any regular medication, or suffer from any chronic medical problem, make sure you discuss your diet plans with your medical practitioner before starting your diet.

6. Set yourself a realistic target and timetable for weight loss (see above). Go slowly but surely.

7. Be aware that the first month of dieting always produces the most rapid weight loss, because the energy stores used up first by the body during a diet contain a lot of water. What is more, as you approach your target weight, your diet becomes relatively less severe in calorie terms, and so weight loss slows down (remember, a person at their ideal weight needs to eat fewer calories each day than they did when they were overweight).

8. Keep as physically active as possible when you are dieting.

9. Enlist all the support you can from friends, family and workmates to make your diet as easy and enjoyable as possible.

10. Remember, you are not simply going on a diet, you are changing your life for the better.

16. *What foods are good for weaning my baby on to solids?*

Weaning is the period between about six months and thirty to thirty-six months (when the first set of teeth have come through) during which a child makes the change from a liquid diet to a diet based on solids. It is a time of great nutritional importance, and there is increasing evidence that good early nutrition helps to prevent disease (especially heart disease) in later life. It also helps to produce a fit and healthy child who grows and gains weight at a normal rate.

Even though the efficiency of breast milk as a complete baby food diminishes a little after six months, there are still emotional and nutritional benefits to be gained from continuing to breast feed (in slowly decreasing amounts) whilst introducing weaning foods. In particular, it gives the baby time to adjust comfortably to the change in diet.

Good weaning foods are those which can be prepared in different consistencies and which supply good amounts of energy and essential nutrients like iron. They should be low in fibre (especially at first) and not highly seasoned. A thin porridge based on a cereal (not wheat) should be tried once a day at first, with feeds slowly getting thicker in consistency and more frequent as the baby gets used to the new flavours and sensations. By eighteen months, a puréed version of the family's normal diet is usually sufficient to provide complete nutrition. Solid foods should continue to be crushed until the first set of teeth is through, at which point weaning ends.

17. *How does naturopathic nutrition apply to childhood and adolescence?*

Families with good diets mean children with good diets, so perhaps the most important aspect of childhood nutrition is the example of the parent/s. It is no good parents preaching good eating habits without having good eating habits themselves.

In Western society, research has shown that dietary deficiency is extremely rare in schoolchildren. The children most likely to be taking nutritional supplements – children with well-off parents – are those least likely to need them, and vitamin and mineral supplements have not been shown to produce any particular benefit in children taking them. The real threat to childhood nutrition is one of excess, especially excess of sugar, fat (particularly saturated fat), cholesterol and salt.

Unfortunately, though most schoolchildren seem to know that some foods are good for you and others bad, they don't choose what they eat on the basis of this knowledge. Lack of dietary example, lack of availability of healthy food, and social pressure driven by advertising are widely regarded as the cause of this.

It is vital, therefore, that the home provides a framework for good nutrition of the child by providing the following:

1. An example of healthy eating set by the parent/s.

2. Good stocks of healthy food that are easily available at home.

3. Regular meal times, with as much time as possible for breakfast.

4. Simple 'food guides' to help children eat well when away from home.

Part of providing a good dietary example is to be aware of the effect of the media, not only on children, but on yourself. In 1977, fifty percent of commercials shown during children's TV programmes in the UK were advertising food products, the majority for sugary or fast foods. The key to healthy food shopping – easy to say but surprisingly hard to do – is don't buy what you don't approve of. If it's not in the house, you won't eat it. If you don't eat it, there is a chance your children won't either.

It is also important not to use food as a reward or as a weapon in dealing with childhood behaviour difficulties. This may require frequent, tactful reminders to relations and friends, but can be an important way of breaking the link between being good and foods high in sugar and fat, but low in nutrition. That is not to say that snacking is unhealthy – as long as the snacks themselves are healthy.

In the Western world, there is an increasing trend towards childhood fatness (obesity) but research suggests that a low level of physical activity amongst children (often related to watching TV) is just as important a cause as too much eating. Since an obese child is still a growing child, what is needed is *fat* loss, not weight loss. The best way to achieve this is to increase the amount of physical activity in the child's life and let her/him grow up 'into' – and so out of – their fatness. Strict calorie-reducing diets for growing children are rarely a good idea.

After infancy, puberty is the most rapid period of growth ever experienced by a human being. Surprisingly, energy needs are only slightly increased during this time, but the developing adolescent requires a diet of high nutritional quality since growth and sexual maturation need proper levels of vitamins, minerals and proteins. In young women, menstruation also raises the dietary requirement for iron.

Of course, puberty does not happen all at once. It is a process which begins with a striking spurt in growth. Girls tend to reach their full adult height earlier than boys and so, although men are (on average) 15cm taller and 15kg heavier than women, during puberty girls are often taller than boys.

Although nutritional deficiencies are rare in adolescence, over-nutrition and dietary imbalance are increasing along with increased levels of alcohol and drug abuse. So the cornerstones of good diet – such as low sugar, low fat, low salt, minimum snacking and regular meal times – are of particular importance to teenagers.

Over- and under-weight can also be very important during adolescence. As with the growing child, dieting during the puberty growth spurt is not recommended, even for obese teenagers. It is far better to tackle the problem by increasing the amount of physical activity, which also improves the development of muscles and bones.

Since eating disorders affect at least one in a hundred young women and many young men in Western society, all parents of adolescents should be aware of the features of anorexia nervosa and bulimia nervosa. These are:

Anorexia

- Refusal to maintain a minimum body weight.

- Fear of gaining weight, despite being underweight.

- Disturbance of perception of body weight/shape.

- For young women, missing three periods.

Bulimia

- Recurrent bingeing (twice a week or more for at least three months).

- Being unable to control binges.
- Regular self-induced vomiting and/or use of laxatives, diuretics, dieting, fasting or vigorous exercise to control weight.
- Persistent concern over body weight and size.

Fanaticism about a high energy sport (swimming, running, etc.) may need help and advice if weight loss becomes a problem. It is also important that any young person wishing to avoid animal products in their diet should understand that vegetarianism is not just about cutting out what you don't want to eat; it is also about eating more of a wider variety of the foods you do want to eat.

18. *How should my diet change as I get older?*

The need for energy decreases to some extent with age, so foods with less calories – but with good concentrations of essential nutrients, such as vegetables and fruits – are particularly suitable. Except in particular cases of disease, dietary deficiencies of vitamins and minerals in old age are rare, and the issue of calcium and osteoporosis has already been discussed in Question 13. Vitamin D deficiency can be a risk, particularly for the bedridden or housebound but, as with other age groups, this can be prevented very effectively by increased exposure to sunlight.

The heart of good nutrition during later years is a simple diet, rich in complex carbohydrates, with a moderate fibre intake from natural sources, a low level of saturated fat and low intake of sugary/starchy foods (to help with oral hygiene). Also, as the human body ages, its water content decreases and the efficiency of the kidneys declines. The elderly person therefore requires more water to be able to excrete waste products, and should drink a reasonable amount of water each day.

Of course, illness and disease may affect the diet of the older person, and many elderly people experience difficulty in purchasing, preparing and cooking food for themselves. However, since good nutrition is a major factor in maintaining a high quality of life – social, physical and psychological – during old age, it should be a priority for all those involved in helping and caring for the elderly. Some help with shopping and food budgeting, a home and kitchen environment appropriate to physical abilities, and care that medication or illness is not interfering with nutrition are all likely to be of more benefit to an older person than vitamin or mineral supplements.

One of Britain's longest lived men, Harry Shoerats (who died in February

1984, aged 111) was a good example of the benefits of naturopathic nutrition. He worked as a craftsman until the age of 104, cycled to work daily until his 100th birthday and attributed his long life and good health primarily to his diet of fruits, nuts, vegetables and cereals.

19. *What special dietary precautions should I take during pregnancy?*

Pregnancy requires a wealth of physical changes and adjustments in the mother's body, the most noticeable of which is weight gain. This weight gain affects energy and nutrient needs, and is also a vital part of the process of producing a healthy baby. A developing baby is in fact responsible for only about a quarter of the weight gained in a normal pregnancy. The rest is made up of extra water in the mother's blood and tissues, plus some extra fat and protein.

Weight gain is slow for the first ten weeks of pregnancy, but increases fairly steadily from this point until birth. Body fat tends to accumulate most rapidly in the middle of pregnancy, usually around the shoulders, upper thighs and abdomen. This fat helps meet the needs of the growing baby and also helps to provide energy for breast feeding. (Breast feeding is therefore a natural way for a mother to lose weight after pregnancy although, since appetite also increases during breast feeding, most women are left with some overall weight gain after each pregnancy.)

The COMA (Committee on Medical Aspects of Food Policy) Report (1991) estimated that, for a 60kg woman, pregnancy requires a total of an extra 67,161 kilocalories (281 megajoules) of energy to support the needs of the mother and the growing baby. However, there is no worldwide agreement on the amount of extra *food* energy necessary during pregnancy to provide this. In affluent Western societies, a general decrease in physical activity during pregnancy (and various other adjustments of the metabolism) mean that it is probably not necessary to eat extra calories each day to support the demands of pregnancy. Most mothers only eat a little more during pregnancy, and this is mostly in the last three months.

Assuming that you are not undernourished at the beginning of pregnancy, COMA recommends that no increase in calorie intake is necessary until the last three months, during which time they suggest an increase of 200 kilocalories per day. However, it is very unwise to go more than six to eight hours without eating at *any* time during pregnancy, since this may interfere with the baby's metabolism.

In the West, where most women consume more than enough protein, it is not usually necessary to recommend a dietary increase to cover the extra

925 grams of protein that are accumulated during pregnancy by the mother and the baby. Nevertheless, the COMA report does recommend a small daily increase in protein intake. The World Health Organisation suggests that any increases are made more in the second and, particularly, the third trimesters.

As far as fats are concerned, a good intake of foods containing alpha-linolenic acid (such as safflower oil, olive oil, sunflower seeds and the various grains) is important, particularly in the last trimester. Alpha-linolenic acid is used by the foetus to produce chemicals vital for normal brain development.

There is no reliable or conclusive evidence that pregnancy changes the need for vitamins and minerals, but various food committees around the world nevertheless suggest increased intakes – by anything from ten to one hundred percent, depending on the committee. Iron deficiency may occur, particularly in teenage mothers, those who have had several children and those suffering the effects of poverty. A poor diet and heavy periods before conception also increase the risk.

Although the growing baby demands a good iron supply to build up its iron reserves prior to birth, a well nourished, healthy mother can obtain all the iron necessary from food (such as parsley, greens, dried fruits, chick-peas and almonds). However, it is important to be aware of the possibility of iron deficiency in pregnancy so that its symptoms (tiredness and breathlessness out of proportion to effort, sometimes palpitations) are recognized and appropriate action taken. (See also page 240.)

There is also evidence that an increase in folate consumption before conception and during the first three months of pregnancy can help reduce the risk of spina bifida and other neural tube defects. As a result, government health departments in many countries now advise all women who are considering having a baby and those who are already pregnant to take a folate supplement (particularly if they have already had a child with a neural tube defect). Good sources of food folate include beans, green vegetables, beetroot and muesli.

Nutritional advice for a healthy pregnancy can be summed up as follows:

- Eat a nourishing diet *before* pregnancy and maintain a good body weight.

- Eat a nourishing diet *during* pregnancy and gain weight at a normal rate.

- Ensure you meet your daily energy needs adequately.

- Don't go for too long between meals.

- Take note of government advice on vitamin supplementation.

20. *Why is breast feeding better than bottle feeding and should I be eating more if I am breast feeding?*

The infant human grows at a remarkable pace, but has a digestive system that cannot tolerate solids, high fibre or toxic substances. It also cannot deal with food that is too concentrated, because its kidneys are immature and must not be overloaded.

Breast milk is, therefore, the perfect food for human babies, particularly for the first four to six months of life. It has a number of features that are impossible to reproduce in manufactured foods, the most striking of which is the change in its composition according to the baby's needs. The colostrum milk, produced during the first five days of breast feeding, is higher in protein, immunoglobulins, cholesterol and important trace elements, such as zinc and selenium. After five days, if the mother is healthy and well nourished herself, the milk changes its composition during each feed and also as the day goes on. One of the components of breast milk, secretory IgA, provides the baby with protection against digestive and respiratory infections by neutralizing toxins and viruses. It may also help to prevent food sensitivities and allergic reactions, which are less common in breast-fed infants.

There has been some research suggesting that breast milk may be insufficient in certain respects (for example in vitamin K, fluoride and, for babies over the age of four months or so, in vitamin D and iron), but such research is hard to interpret because there is such a great variation between mothers in the composition of their milk at any given time. What is more, one of the potential breast milk deficiencies is easily remedied. A fully clothed baby, not wearing a hat, needs only to be out in daylight (preferably sunshine) for about two hours each week to be able to make sufficient vitamin D for good health. (See pages 89–90 for information on vitamin D and sunlight.)

The successful survival of the human race for thousands of years before the discovery of vitamins is in itself sufficient testimony to the adequacy of human breast milk.

Cow's milk contains too much protein for baby kidneys to cope with, and is low in a number of essential nutrients (such as linoleic acid and niacin). So it has to be chemically manipulated and supplemented to make adequate baby formulas. Moreover, there is always the possibility of a baby becoming allergic to cow proteins and also, after a bout of gastroenteritis, to milk sugar (lactose). Of course, formula foods have improved greatly over the years, but knowledge of infant nutritional needs is far from complete even today. As a result, formulae keep being revised and changed by manufacturers.

The manufacture of cow's milk formulae also carries social and environmental costs and, given the amount of baby milk exported to the Third

World, it is deeply disturbing to realize that it is more expensive to provide formula milk for undernourished babies than it is to feed undernourished mothers to a level where they can produce sufficient breast milk to feed their babies themselves. Even worse, it has been estimated that, to date, more than nine million babies have died from drinking cow's milk formulae made up with infected water in countries suffering the effects of poverty.

After about four months of age, it is sometimes said that the 'non-nutritional advantages' of breast feeding – such as the bonding between mother and baby, and the fact that there is little risk of breast milk becoming contaminated or infected – become less important; many babies are therefore changed to formula feeds (or are given supplementary bottle feeds) around this time. However, the fact that bottle-fed or supplemented babies tend to gain weight faster than breast milk only babies does not, in itself, mean that formula foods are a good thing – except in cases where it is not possible to breast feed.

Goat's milk and sheep's milk have no particular advantage over cow's milk as the basis of formula foods. The only advantage of soya milk formulae is that, since they contain no milk sugar (lactose), they are useful for babies with lactose intolerance. Soya-derived milk is, of course, very different from human milk and, like cow's milk, requires supplementation and alteration to become an acceptable food for babies. On the other hand, it is arguably no worse than cow's milk. Although public concern over aluminium levels in soya formulas is justifiable, cow's milk baby formulae and weaning foods are also worrying in this respect. Reports dating back to 1986 show that aluminium levels in many brands of baby food are unacceptably high.

The short answer to good infant nutrition is to breast feed whenever possible. Good nutrition for the mother is vitally important for maintaining the health of the baby, since a well-nourished mother is more likely to be able to breast feed successfully. Where breast feeding is not possible, modern low-aluminium formula feeds provide a good alternative.

Breast milk is a high energy food, and a mother requires extra energy to help her body make the average of 750ml of milk per day that she produces during the first four to six months of breast feeding. To provide this energy, an extra 400 to 450 kcals per day are needed from food, which simply means eating a bit more than usual.

Apart from this, the nutritional needs of breast feeding can be met by eating an adequate amount of healthy food and getting out into the daylight for a few hours each week. Recommendations to increase protein and other nutrient intakes during lactation are based more on assumption than evidence. For example, breast feeding uses up about 210 milligrams of calcium each day during the first six months, but there is no conclusive evidence linking this to bone problems in mothers. Iron needs during breast feeding are much lower than in pregnancy – lower, in fact, than during menstruation – so there is no need to increase iron intake either.

A baby's need for extra vitamin K is the subject of much discussion. Because newborn babies' vitamin K levels do not appear to be high enough to protect them from the small risk of developing Haemolytic Disease of the Newborn (HDN)[12], they used to be given a single injection of vitamin K at birth to boost their reserves. However, vitamin K injections are no longer recommended since there is some evidence that they may be associated with an increased risk of childhood cancer. The effectiveness of giving newborn infants vitamin K by mouth to prevent HDN is still under debate.

Pesticide and pollutant contaminated foods, drugs, alcohol and smoking all decrease the quality and the quantity of milk produced during lactation. On the other hand, good nutrition during pregnancy and a healthy, high-energy diet during breast feeding help to ensure the well-being of both mother and baby.

---

[12]Babies need vitamin K for their blood clotting mechanisms to work properly. If they are lacking in vitamin K, they may develop internal bleeding, particularly within the brain, which may prove fatal. This condition is rare.

CHAPTER NINE

TREATING ILLNESS BY PROMOTING HEALTH

This chapter describes naturopathic concepts of health and disease and explains the principles of natural balance which underlie the use of diet in the treatment of illness.

Natural forces, natural balance

We live in a world of constant change where the strong survive, a world in which failure to adapt means extinction. The human race has lasted so long on the earth because of its ability to respond to change, an ability which is based on the self-healing force: vitality. To understand the relationship between health, disease and survival, we need to understand in practical terms how vitality works. To understand vitality, we have only to look at nature.

Nature has a remarkable ability to maintain a sustainable overall balance between all things at all times, and it achieves this by the operation of three fundamental natural forces:

The Creative Force
The Destructive Force
The Preserving Force

The Creative Force is the tendency to convert energy into matter and is seen in the plant as it converts sunlight into food, in the lioness as she uses the energy of an antelope's flesh to produce milk for her cubs; and in the factory as it turns the energy of coal and gas into machines and materials.

The Destructive Force is the tendency to convert matter into energy, and is seen wherever dead tissue and waste material is decomposed by micro-organisms back into earth; wherever food is digested and turned into energy for movement; and wherever fuel is burnt for heat and light.

The Preserving Force acts to maintain optimum conditions for life, and preserves balance, both between and within natural systems. Whilst its operation may not be so obvious as the other two forces, when you observe nature closely it becomes clear that adjustments are constantly being made which maintain the ecosystem as a whole in a state of balance, a balance that allows maximum life and maximum diversity. For example, the sea keeps an exact and constant concentration of salts in its water, despite the huge seasonal changes in the amount of fresh water pouring into it from rivers.

If the Creative and Destructive forces were left to themselves, there would still be balance of a sort in nature, but not necessarily a balance favouring life, evolution and variety. The Preserving Force acts as the ombudsman between the Creative and the Destructive Forces, making sure that neither gets out of hand. It is the pivot on which the see-saw of life balances.

Nevertheless, it is important to realize that the three fundamental forces in nature are all *equally* important. Without the Destructive Force to break down dead material, there would be no energy to fuel the creation of new life forms by the Creative Force. Without the Preserving Force, there would be no balance between acts of creation and acts of destruction.

Vitality – the nuts and bolts

The three fundamental forces can also be seen to be working within us and together they produce the self-healing capacity known as vitality or life force. In other words, vitality is the operation of the three fundamental forces of nature within living beings.

The Creative Force – which can also be called 'anabolism' – drives the process in which the energy from food is used to combine simple chemical compounds into arms, legs, livers, lungs and other tissues. Put simply, it makes bodies out of food. It makes us grow from child to adult, builds up our reserves and repairs us when we are broken. The Creative Force works most effectively during times of rest and relaxation.

The Destructive Force, or 'catabolism', converts our food (and, when necessary, energy stored in our tissues) into the energy we need to walk, talk and get on with our lives. In other words, it converts food into activity. It helps us rid our bodies of waste materials and enables us to mobilize energy quickly when we need to remove ourselves from situations that may cause us harm.

The Preserving Force, or 'homoeostasis', tries to maintain optimum conditions for health, whatever the changes in circumstance. It keeps our heart beating at an appropriate rate, maintains our blood pressure and keeps the composition of our blood as constant as the sea keeps its salts. This force makes sure our body is neither too acid nor too alkaline, keeps our internal body temperature constant, whether we are in Alaska or Africa, and adjusts our breathing so that there is always the right amount of oxygen available to our tissues. Homoeostasis ensures that all necessary adjustments are made to keep balance within the body as a whole, by keeping balance between anabolic and catabolic processes.

As in nature, all three fundamental forces are equally necessary and equally good for us. Without the Creative and Destructive Forces breaking down and building up tissues according to need, we would not be able to adapt to the constantly changing world. But to survive the process of continual adaptation, we must keep our internal environment as constant as possible, and this is achieved by the Preserving Force.

So our vitality, though it has three faces, is really just one thing: our fundamental capacity to adapt to change. The greater our vitality, the greater our capacity to adapt, and the healthier we are. From this perspective, health is a state of dynamic balance between us and our surroundings. In health, we keep a balance between work and rest, and are able to adapt to and cope with the stresses of life. There is time to play and enjoy life without worry. We have time to appreciate ourselves as a part of the wonder of nature, with our role to play in the evolution of life.

The most important thing about understanding how vitality operates, however, is that it gives us a simple way of dealing with illness, a way to treat disease by encouraging health.

The nature of illness

One of the things that often surprises students of medicine is the realization that the symptoms and signs of illness are not actually caused by diseases, but are caused by the body's attempts to restore normality in the face of unusual circumstances. When you shut your finger in a door, the initial pain encourages you to get your finger out of the door. The subsequent swelling, redness, heat and discomfort are the result of the body reacting to the presence of damaged tissue by trying to heal it. Without inflammation, wounded tissues do not heal.

When bacteria or viruses multiply in our bodies, the immune system may react by trying to get rid of them. But it is the fall-out from this internal chemical warfare that causes the main features of infection, not the organisms themselves.

When we smoke, the lining of the bronchial tubes of our lungs changes in order to make the lungs more resistant to the worst effects of the smoke. Unfortunately, this tougher lining makes the smoker more prone to other lung problems, such as bronchitis. A continuing attempt at self-protection by the bronchial cells may even lead to cancer formation. In other words, smoker's cough, bronchitis and lung cancer are all caused by the body trying to protect itself from smoke.

To summarize, when our reactions to changes in circumstance cause internal imbalance, we become ill in order to restore internal balance. There is therefore only one disease: imbalance.

The wheel of health

Like all other living organisms, we have certain basic requirements for continuing life. These are food, rest and activity. If we eat unadulterated natural food when we're hungry, stop when we're satisfied, drink when we're thirsty, rest when we're tired and move when we feel active, the natural forces within us will be in balance and we will feel healthy (see Diagram 1a).

If we eat or drink too much or too little, push ourselves too far when we are tired, or take too little or too much exercise, the balance of our internal

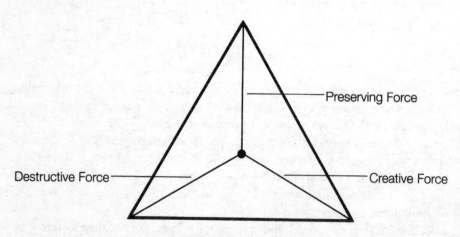

Diagram 1a   The balance of natural forces in health.

forces will alter in order to remedy the situation. And, since doing anything about anything requires energy, the first internal reaction is always an increase in activity of the Destructive Force to make some energy available for change. However, homoeostasis always acts to keep the total amount of energy in the body constant, so this initial catabolic reaction necessarily produces a decrease in the activity of the Creative and Preserving Forces. The resulting imbalance is experienced as illness (see Diagram 1b).

In response to this imbalance, the Preserving (homeostatic) Force gives some of its energy to the Creative (anabolic) Force, so that the Creative and Destructive Forces can come into a new balance with each other. This partial restoration of overall balance is perceived as an improvement in the condition and the increased activity of the Creative (anabolic) and Destructive (catabolic) Forces enables healing to take place (see Diagram 1c).

Although this process of restoring a balance between the Creative and Destructive Forces allows tissues to heal, it also causes a decrease in the Preserving Force. So, during the healing phase of any illness, there is always a susceptibility to further illness, because there is less balancing energy available to cope with any change that may occur in the activity of the other two forces. For this reason, it is extremely important that the period of healing is followed by a period of convalescence, during which the energy of the Preserving Force is restored by the gradual return to normal activity of the Creative and Destructive Forces (see Diagram 1d).

The operation of this system goes more or less unnoticed by us most of the time, just as a car usually runs without us being aware of its mechanical

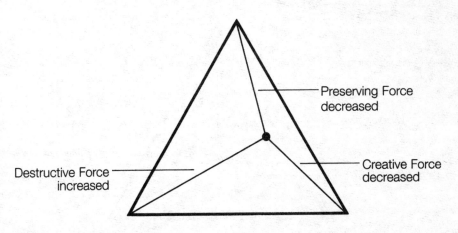

Diagram 1b The imbalance of natural forces during illness.

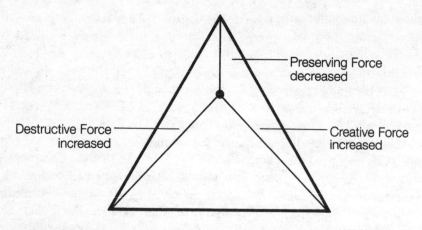

Diagram I c The partial balance of natural forces during healing.

workings. Though small stresses occur, the resulting internal imbalances cause us no particular problems. But, as the day nears its end, accumulated internal imbalance produces a sense of tiredness which, in the end, leads to sleep. During sleep, vitality has a free hand to re-balance and repair our bodies, minds and emotions.

If unrelieved stress starts to become a daily habit, minor symptoms like tiredness, occasional headaches, mild depression and non-specific digestive disturbances begin to occur more often, as the capacity of our vitality to maintain a state of balance between us and our environment is exceeded. In

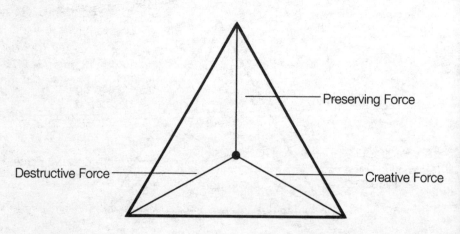

Diagram I d The balance of natural forces restored after convalescence.

these circumstances, acute self-limiting illnesses (colds, 'flu, gastroenteritis, etc.) also occur more frequently, as we try to gain more time for the natural forces to heal and re-balance.

From the discussion and diagrams on the previous pages, it is clear that even minor illnesses deserve a proper period of convalescence to allow time for homoeostasis to regain its full efficiency. Sadly, many people return their shoulder to the wheel at the first opportunity after illness. This may cause no obvious problems for some months (even years), but, if the pattern continues, a sense of deep tiredness or exhaustion starts to become a major feature of daily life. At this point, a period of prolonged rest or relaxation is vitally necessary to restore inner balance; without it, chronic illness of some sort will develop.

If the symptoms of the chronic illness are merely suppressed by medical treatment, and no attempt is made to allow time and space for recovery (which may, at this stage, take several months and a big readjustment in lifestyle), internal imbalance may become so severe that the Destructive Force makes an all or nothing attempt at recovery by producing a major system failure – a heart attack, stroke, cancer or psychotic breakdown, for example. Such extreme circumstances usually result in an enforced period of complete rest during which, bit by bit, tissues heal and vitality is restored. In some cases, however, even this chance to heal is ignored and old, harmful patterns of life are re-established as quickly as possible (but now with the capacity to adapt to change even further reduced than before).

For a few people, of course, the last ditch attempt at true healing creates such extreme imbalance that the forces of nature striving for universal equilibrium take over. At this point, the Destructive Force decomposes tissue back into its basic components, so that the Creative Force can build new life forms once more. Nothing is ever lost. There is truly no death, only change.

In summary, health is successful adaptation to a constantly changing life. It is maintained by our vitality, a self-balancing system of natural forces operating both in nature and within ourselves. If the way we live overstretches the capacity of this system to keep us in internal balance, we experience symptoms of illness as vitality tries to create circumstances suitable for healing (Phase 1 illness). If we allow ourselves proper time for recovery, we will help to ensure that we remain in generally good health, and occasional illness simply becomes part of our normal self-healing process.

On the other hand, if we consistently push ourselves beyond our true capacity to adapt, we risk the development of exhaustion and chronic disease (Phase 2 illness).

If, at this stage, we still fail to rest and recover, we will experience a crisis condition of some sort (Phase 3 illness), which leads to a period of enforced rest, producing either a full recovery, additional chronic symptoms or death.

The relationship between these three phases of illness is illustrated in the following diagram.

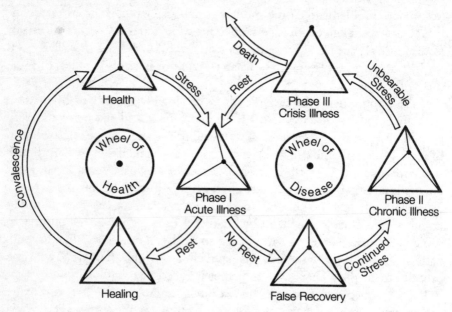

The three phases of illness.

The importance of these concepts is that they provide the basis of a logical, safe and simple self-help strategy for health. Since we don't have diseases, simply imbalances which make us feel ill, if we can restore balance we will get better – whatever our condition is called. If we understand how our lives have produced our particular illness, we can use simple methods to hasten a return to our normal state – health.

Treating illness by promoting health

If we find ourselves suffering illness, the first step in helping ourselves is to recognize where we are on the wheels of health and disease, as illustrated above.

In Phase 1 illness:

1. The person affected is **generally fit** and well and not usually prone to illness (any more than **the average**).

2. The disease is acute, **starting** suddenly, often with fever, sweating and loss of appetite in the early **stages**.

3. The cause is usually obvious – eg. exposure to extremes of climate, exposure to sudden unusual stress, contact with someone else suffering the same condition, a minor accident, etc.

Most acute infections, inflammations, and minor illnesses belong to this phase.

Illness in Phase 2 has the following features:

1. It affects people who have been subjected to a period of physical, mental, emotional or spiritual stress in various combinations and who are constantly tired and run-down, with repeated bouts of minor illness and time off work.

2. It produces 'diseases' that are chronic, with a slow, insidious onset and ill-defined symptoms and signs.

3. The original cause may be in the past, or not very obvious.

4. Treatments tried bring only temporary relief.

Most chronic diseases – both physical and mental – fall into this category eg. angina, asthma, arthritis, migraine, depression, benign tumours like fibroids, stomach ulcers, inflammatory bowel diseases, fungal infections, eczema and psoriasis.

Illness in Phase 3 has the following features:

1. The person affected is in acute crisis, often with a background of chronic imbalance stretching back over many years.

2. The disease involves the failure of a major organ, system or life strategy.

3. The acute features of the crisis condition are made worse by the poor general condition of the person.

Heart attack, acute heart failure, stroke, malignant cancers, kidney failure, liver failure, respiratory failure and serious accidents and poisonings fall into this category.

Having decided which category our illness falls into, we can then start doing things that will help us get well.

Firstly, we can accept that we are where we are, and start working towards a solution from there. We cannot change the past but, if we are alive, something is working and it can often be helped to work better if we start to appreciate what is positive in our situation. Of course, it can be difficult not to worry when illness comes but, if we look at illness as nature's way of giving us the opportunity to regain our health instead of as some sort of retribution or undeserved fate, we can turn our worries into positive steps which help to encourage the healing process.

Secondly, since health depends on balance between the natural forces, the treatment of any illness must:

1. Create circumstances which maximize the beneficial effects of the fundamental natural forces.

2. Remove any internal and external factors that produce continuing or additional stress.

3. Encourage the recovery of full vitality by allowing proper convalescence, however minor the illness.

In Phase 1 illness, the best way to achieve these objectives is to give the body complete peace and rest, whilst making sure that any reaction to the healing process, such as fever, does not get out of hand. Since food requires digesting before its energy can be used, and since digestion requires energy, it is more efficient to allow the body to use its own energy reserves to fuel the healing process than to overload the digestion with food; in other words, it is best not to eat.[1] Illnesses in this phase don't last very long, and almost everyone has some energy reserve stored in their fat. (Catabolic diets suitable for acute Phase 1 conditions are described in detail in Chapter Ten, pages 121–135.)

From the body's point of view, illnesses in Phase 2 result from circumstances similar to driving a car with the accelerator hard down and the clutch only half engaged. We use tablets, treatments and will-power to keep ourselves going – despite feeling near enough worn out – and our body tries to keep the situation under control by releasing steroid hormones from the adrenal glands to damp down our inflammatory and immune reactions, and give us temporary relief. Once again, complete rest and relaxation are vital for real cure, which may take some weeks or even months in some cases. In addition, the depleted energy stores need refilling in a way which doesn't

[1] It is, of course, important to keep an adequate intake of fluids.

demand too much work. In this situation, an easily digested anabolic diet, full of vital energy is needed. (Anabolic diets are described in detail in Chapter Eleven, pages 136–148.)

Illnesses in Phase 3 occur when all available resources have been used up, without the basic problems being solved. The system becomes 'insolvent' and can't manage even basic maintenance. Vitality is so compromised that additional problems like secondary infections may compound the crisis.

Dealing with such conditions requires expert nursing and medical management around the clock, and nutritional strategies cannot be applied until the crisis passes. However, once some basic stability returns, anabolic diets (as described in Chapter Eleven) can be used to speed and improve the healing process, and help maximize the potential for true recovery.

Conclusion

We have seen that, in health, our vitality maintains us in a state of balance and individuality by constantly adjusting the actions of the fundamental forces within us, according to our circumstances. When illness occurs, therefore, we should do everything we can to encourage the restoration of this balance – and as little as possible to disturb it.

In principle, since health in nature and health in us both depend on the same natural forces, all we have to do to treat illness effectively is to use nature's methods. These consist of good and appropriate nourishment, and a proper balance between rest and activity in order to encourage healing.

The problem is that we rarely pay attention these days to our inner sense of what we really need to be well because, until something goes seriously wrong, most of us feel that our capacity to adapt to life's weary stage is unlimited, particularly if we enjoy or gain from the things that put us out of balance and at risk of illness. How often have we *known* that we should get more rest and more exercise, eat better food, drink or smoke less, in order to get well, and yet completely ignored our own advice?[2]

For most of us, for most of our lives, not listening to our inner voice causes few problems. But, as time goes by, if we allow accumulated imbalance to persist, we put ourselves at real risk of illness. This is because vitality always acts to regain a proper balance between the natural forces working within us – whatever the apparent cost – because that is the only way to sustain life in the long term.

[2]We have lost count of the number of times people who are ill, when asked what they think would do them the most good, have said to us 'taking a good long rest …'.

We were born to be healthy. Whatever sort of mind or body nature has given us, it is always possible to live in a state of greater ease of body, mind, emotions and spirit by working with the natural forces, rather than against them. By understanding the fundamental process of illness, and recognizing our own relationship to it, we can use simple methods to restore harmony when illness brings disease. The remainder of Part Three explains how to do this.

CHAPTER TEN

LESS IS MORE

This chapter is about the use of catabolic diets in the treatment of acute illness, and the use of fasting as a general aid to good health. It is not about slimming or weight reduction. Before trying any of the regimes described, it is important that you should read the whole chapter, paying particular attention to the section headed 'Are catabolic diets suitable for everyone?'

When animals are unwell, they stop eating and the same is usually true of humans. In fact, loss of appetite is a major symptom of many acute human diseases. The return of the desire to eat after illness is usually taken as a sign of healing.

Following nature's lead, therefore, people across the centuries have used fasting and dietary restriction to treat all sorts of illness. In ancient Egypt, fasting was recommended as a treatment for diseases such as syphilis and gonorrhoea. The pre-Christian Essene community routinely used dietary restriction as a way of maintaining good health. Even today, health spas offering controlled diets remain popular with those seeking an antidote to the stresses of modern life.

A catabolic diet allows some of the energy normally used for digesting food to be applied to the process of getting well and helps the body to focus its attention on repair and rejuvenation during acute illness (and sometimes during recovery from a chronic illness). Afterwards, the body is able to absorb nutrients from food more effectively and to deal more efficiently with waste materials.

Are catabolic diets suitable for everyone?

Catabolic diets are used mostly to treat acute disease, and are a systematic way of encouraging our natural tendency not to eat when feeling unwell.

They are therefore suitable for the treatment of Phase 1 illness (see Chapter Nine, pages 115–118).

If you are generally well and active for your age, and not suffering from any chronic disease, you can safely choose any of the six catabolic diets described below to help you recover efficiently from acute Phase 1 disturbances, such as colds, 'flus, simple infections, food poisonings, minor digestive disturbances and uncomplicated strains, sprains, accidents and anxieties. The advantage of catabolic dieting over conventional symptom suppression in these circumstances is that you will make a true, rather than partial recovery. By eliminating stored up toxins, you will finish your illness noticeably healthier and more energetic than you were when it began.

If you have an established, but stable (and untroublesome) chronic condition, and would like to use catabolic dieting to help you deal with occasional minor illness, you should follow one of the milder regimes (such as catabolic diets 1 or 2).

Children and adolescents are normally self-regulating when it comes to food and illness and they should be allowed to be so. Catabolic dieting is not therefore recommended for those under 18 years of age, except on the advice of a registered naturopath (see page 253 for a list of helpful addresses). However, catabolic diet 1 can be a useful first-aid measure for older children at the first sign of a cold or other minor upper respiratory tract infection.

Do not undertake catabolic diets at times in your life where you need to build up your tissues, such as during pregnancy[1], breast feeding or times of immobilization after accidents or major operations. People suffering from serious chronic disease, anorexia or bulimia should not use catabolic diets at all.

If you are on any sort of medication, do not start catabolic dieting without first consulting your health care practitioner. People who are very overweight should not go on a catabolic diet without the supervision of a registered naturopath.

Although mainly used to speed recovery from acute Phase 1 conditions, catabolic diets also have a use in the treatment of chronic Phase 2 illness, but only when recovery is well underway and there is sufficient energy available to cope with increased tissue breakdown and the elimination of toxins. Since a catabolic diet uses up stored energy, a certain level of vitality has to be reached before starting one (in the same way that it is impossible to bump start a car with no battery, however much fuel there is in the tank). The time

[1]Morning sickness in early pregnancy can sometimes be much relieved by a short period of gentle catabolic dieting, however.

to use a catabolic diet during recovery from chronic disease is discussed in the next chapter.

Phase 3 or crisis illness often produces an enforced fast because of its severity in the acute stage but, as we noted in Chapter Nine, the management of such illness requires expert help and guidance.

Catabolic diets: the principles

The natural instinct to stop eating when we are ill is based on three biological principles:

1. The process of digesting food and absorbing, metabolizing and storing nutrients requires a lot of energy. Restricting food intake during illness allows some of this energy to be channelled into the process of healing and repair.

2. When the body is denied food from the outside, it breaks down its own substance, particularly fatty tissue, to provide energy. This tissue breakdown is not indiscriminate, however. When external food sources are restricted, the body decomposes and burns diseased, damaged, old and dead cells, and tissues first, in the same way that predators in the wild will hunt and eat old and weak animals first, thus ensuring the health of the flock as a whole.

3. When toxins, poisons or allergic substances enter the body at a rate greater than it is able to deal with straightaway, they are stored – walled-off so to speak – in fatty tissue (or bone) where they will do no harm. Using up excess fat stores by restricting food intake helps to remove stored toxins from the body.

These three principles form the basis of all catabolic diets.

Catabolic diets involve reducing food intake at the first sign of acute illness. Research has shown that when the burden of digestion is removed from the body, the organs responsible for getting rid of waste products (the kidneys, liver, lungs and skin) work more efficiently; and, for the average Westerner, blood levels of sugar and protein remain quite normal even during a severely restricted diet. Since the body has an astonishing ability to discriminate between essential and non-essential tissues, our vital organs, glands and nervous tissues are not 'digested' or damaged during a catabolic diet; it is the diseased, aged and dead tissues that are broken down and used for fuel. What is more, catabolic diets do not have to be severe to be useful; several of the regimes discussed below are very gentle and allow unrestricted intake of a variety of healthy foods.

Overall, catabolic diets increase the rate of tissue repair and renewal in the body and, at the same time, allow the removal of accumulated toxic or harmful substances. In this respect, you can imagine the body as a 'sorting office' in which incoming letters are sorted into useful mail and junk-mail. If there is an excessive amount of junk-mail, the system starts to clog up and break down. A person who over-eats, or has a diet containing too much non-nutritious junk food, has too much incoming junk-mail and risks pushing their body towards an unbalanced, diseased state. However, if the situation is not too advanced, reducing the 'incoming mail' by going on a catabolic diet allows the system to throw out the junk, clear the backlog and get back to normal working.

Types of catabolic diet

There are six main types of catabolic diet:

1. The raw fruit and cooked/raw vegetable diet with rice.
2. The raw fruit and cooked/raw vegetable diet.
3. The raw fruit and vegetable diet.
4. The mixed fruit diet.
5. The mono-fruit diet.
6. The total fast.

Before discussing the practical aspects of catabolic dieting, we will describe each one in turn so that you can get a feel for what is involved.

1. The raw fruit and cooked/raw vegetable diet with rice

In this diet, you eat as much as you like, as often as you like, of the following:

a. Fresh vegetables, raw and/or cooked, chosen from groups 1, 2, 3, 4, 5, 6a(i), 6a(ii), and 7a (see pages 32–34 for lists of the different food groups).

b. Fresh raw fruits and berries chosen from groups 7b, 7c and 8 (see page 34).

You can also eat up to three portions of boiled rice (brown or white) per day.
   Organic produce is best (but not essential), and it may be advisable to keep off the Solanaceae family of vegetable (potatoes, tomatoes, aubergines and peppers), since these can sometimes provoke food allergy. You should drink spring water whenever you are thirsty.

Catabolic diet 1 is a gentle, cleansing regime which avoids rapid breakdown of energy stores, and so avoids any strong reactions.

2. The raw fruit and cooked/raw vegetable diet

This is the same as diet 1, except that you leave out the rice. Eat as much as you like, as often as you like, of all sorts of fresh vegetables (raw or cooked according to preference) and fresh, raw fruits, and drink spring water according to thirst. Being slightly lower in calories than diet 1, the elimination of waste products and toxins from the body is more rapid.

3. The raw fruit and vegetable diet

In the raw fruit and vegetable diet, you choose any fresh fruits and vegetables you like and eat them raw, whenever you want. Choose from food groups 1, 2, 3, 4, 5, 7a, 7b, 7c and 8, plus fresh peas and sprouts from group 6 (see pages 32–35). Once again, it may be advisable to keep off the Solanaceae family of vegetables (potatoes, tomatoes, aubergines and peppers).

You should eat as your hunger dictates, but only raw fruits and vegetables. Drink spring water according to thirst. Organic vegetables are preferable, but don't be put off if you can't get them. It is still better to do the diet using non-organic vegetables than not to do it at all.

4. The mixed fruit diet

The mixed fruit diet is based on any mixture of fruits from groups 7b and 7c (see page 34) that suits your taste. Eat your favourite fruits – as much of them as you like and when you like – and drink spring water when you are thirsty. If available, organic fruit improves the quality of the diet.

Fruits contain a lot of water, are easily digested and consist mainly of carbohydrates that are easy to use for fuel (ie. disaccharides). Most fruits also have a very high vitamin C content, which encourages tissue healing and is a natural antioxidant and a good laxative. Orange/yellow coloured fruits also usually contain beta-carotene, another important anti-oxidant vitamin. The non-starch polysaccharide (fibre) in fruit, particularly the soluble pectin, is of proven benefit to health.

Certain fruits have particular beneficial properties. Papaya and pineapple, for example, contain enzymes which aid the process of digestion. Bananas have a high content of potassium, which can be useful in the relief of gastroenteritis and diarrhoea.

5. The mono-fruit diet

In the mono-fruit diet, you choose just one variety of fruit from group 7b (see page 34) to eat throughout. You can eat as much as you like of your chosen fruit and drink pure water according to your thirst. Grapes are one of the fruits suitable for the mono-fruit diet, especially at the end of the summer when they are cheap and plentiful. You can use any fruit you like for a mono-fruit diet, however, as long as it is a fruit that 'agrees with you'.

6. The total fast

In a traditional total fast, the only substance that passes the lips is spring or mineral water. However, some people find it more acceptable to include diluted fruit juices (eg. apple or grape) and/or vegetable juices diluted half and half with spring or mineral water. You can drink as much as you like on a total fast, but a minimum of eight glasses (ie. 1.5 litres) of fluid should be drunk each day.

Practical catabolic dieting

If you would like to try one of the catabolic diets described above, here is a checklist to guide you through the process:

1. *Whilst you are well, decide which of the six diets is likely to suit you best.*

If, in the event, you feel the chosen diet does not suit you for any reason, you can always change to another one, or even stop.

2. *Prepare yourself mentally for the process of catabolic dieting.*

The length and severity of a catabolic diet is always in your control. Bear in mind, though, that any initial increase in hunger will almost certainly diminish after the first couple of days as the body switches over to 'internal combustion'. It is worth persevering early on.

Also, catabolic diets sometimes produce what is known as a 'healing crisis' and this needs to be recognized and understood. The healing crisis and its benefits are explained later in the chapter.

Most important, don't underestimate the power of a positive mental attitude in recovery from illness. The beneficial effects of a catabolic diet will last well beyond the illness itself, and there is great satisfaction to be gained from taking some responsibility for your own health.

3. *At the first sign of an acute illness, find a peaceful, warm environment where you can get as much rest as you need, when you need it.*

Catabolic diets are about using all your available resources for healing and repair, so it is vital to get plenty of rest. It is also important to avoid getting cold, because getting cold means using up energy to get warm again.

4. *Start your chosen diet and stick to it.*

It is not easy to be precise about how long to continue a catabolic diet since its effect will depend on the severity of the illness, the amount of energy you have available for healing and the time you are prepared to allow yourself off from work or normal daily activities.

In general, if you have chosen one of catabolic diets 1 to 5, continue dieting until your symptoms disappear completely (up to a maximum of two weeks for diets 1, 2 and 3, and 12 days for diets 4 and 5). You can then start the return to normal eating, introducing extra foods one at a time with tea, coffee, alcohol, dairy products and meats added last. Remember that a return of real, enthusiastic hunger after a period of catabolic dieting is usually a sign that healing has taken place.

If you have decided on diet 6, a total fast, do not continue with it for more than three days, except on the advice of a registered naturopath. (See list of useful addresses at the end of the book.) You could, however, continue with one of the less stringent diets until you feel entirely well.

In all cases, if your symptoms have not started to diminish after three days, consider getting advice from a suitably qualified health professional. If you are not completely well after a fortnight, or your symptoms recur after having passed through a healing crisis, you should also seek the advice of a competent practitioner.

5. *Drink water, little and often.*

The water you drink during a catabolic diet should be as pure as possible, which probably means buying bottled spring/mineral water. Drink as much as your thirst dictates (you will probably get through at least a bottle a day) and remember that for all the liquid that comes out of your body, some more has to go in to replace it.

Sweating, breathing fast, diarrhoea and passing large amounts of urine are all ways of losing water from the body; in these circumstances, make sure that you are drinking enough to balance the losses. You may be surprised how much better drinking little and often can make you feel during an acute illness.

6. *Allow yourself a period of convalescence equal to the number of days that you were ill before returning to normal activity.*

It is essential to allow an appropriate length of time for convalescence. Failure to do so is storing up trouble for the future; a few extra days back at work now will not compensate for the possible months (or years) of chronic illness – or the weeks spent recovering from a major crisis – that can result when simple illness is repeatedly not allowed proper time to heal. However, convalescence doesn't mean staying in bed. Gentle exercise, time spent in the fresh air or enjoying a non-strenuous hobby, etc. can all help the process of true recovery.

7. *If you are a smoker, we strongly advise you to abstain from smoking while on a catabolic diet.*

Smoking may make you feel even more unwell, and it diminishes the quality of the diet.

8. *No alcohol should be consumed during a catabolic diet.*

Alcohol puts an unnecessary extra strain on the liver and kidneys.

What to expect

If you use catabolic diets to deal with acute illness, it is clearly important to recognize the effects the diets themselves are having on your body, so that you can feel confident they are helping you towards full recovery.

The effects of catabolic diets can be listed under four headings:

- Minor effects
- Healing crises
- The re-surfacing of old problems
- After-effects

Minor effects

As already described, one of the main effects of catabolic diets is to increase the rate of elimination of waste materials from the body in the urine, faeces, sweat and breath. So it is not uncommon for the urine to appear a little darker and to have a stronger odour, for the bowels to become looser, for sweating to increase and for the breath to smell slightly unpleasant during the first couple of days. The tongue may also appear coated. Some degree of increased tiredness is inevitable as the body is working hard to heal itself.

Healing crises

The concept of the healing crisis is as old as medicine itself, and all medical professionals have had the experience of a patient's condition getting a little worse just before it gets very much better. However, significant healing crises are unlikely to occur on the mild or short-term catabolic diets described above. They are more usually experienced during total fasts, undertaken for their 'natural spring cleaning' effects (see page 130).

Re-surfacing of old problems

Since catabolic diets encourage the removal of old, diseased or damaged tissue from the body, it is not uncommon to experience a brief recurrence of an old problem during longer diets. A young woman in our care went on a total fast; during that time, she had an abnormal menstrual period in which some old, foul-smelling blood and tissue was passed. She had experienced a miscarriage some years earlier, and had always felt something had been 'left behind'. When she started using her own tissues to provide energy during the fast, the old 'walled off' material was dissolved and the problem released. She has had no problems with her periods since.

After-effects

The main after-effect of catabolic dieting, rest and proper convalescence is a feeling of positive health and well-being. The mind is alert, the emotions peaceful and the body vigorous. Breath is fresh, the urine is light and not strong smelling, and the bowels are regular and calm. Best of all, the ability to cope with life and avoid illness is increased.

The experience of a catabolic diet may alter your view of food quite substantially. Foods previously much liked may lose their attraction, and new patterns of eating may establish themselves. After a catabolic diet, it is easier to 'hear' what your body is telling you about which foods are best to eat and which are better avoided.

Natural spring-cleaning

In every home, it is occasionally necessary to clear out the food cupboard because, if old food accumulates, it will eventually go stale and create problems. It may attract mice or flies, or it may become infected with harmful bacteria. Food may go mouldy or the smell may become unpleasant. Cleaning up the food cupboard is a basic part of good house keeping. It involves throwing out things that have gone too far past their sell-by date, using up or composting left-overs and sorting the fresh from the old.

Similarly, fasting during health can be used to clear the body of accumulated debris and to reduce long term susceptibility to stress and illness. It is a particularly good preventive health measure, since the average modern Western diet contains so many toxins in the form of hormones, antibiotics, pesticides, herbicides, preservatives and colorants, in addition to empty calories and too much fat. This slow but constant ingestion of substances that disturb the body's natural function and balance may even be related to diseases of the immune system (such as auto-immune conditions and allergies).

So a fast, undertaken when you are feeling fit and have some time to devote to yourself, is a good way of giving your body a chance to do some serious spring-cleaning. It allows everything that has been pushed to the back of the cupboard during busy times to be cleaned out.

Traditionally, fasting was done during spring, a time when we all feel a natural urge to clean, repair and renew our surroundings. Cleansing tonics, such as birch juice, were drunk, and a catabolic diet consisting only of the green shoots of dandelion and other plants high in vitamins, but low in calories, would be followed.

The stringencies of Ramadan and the forty day fast of Lent are other examples of catabolic dieting. Religious fasting is thus not only an act of praise to an external God, but also a way to praise and honour God within ourselves.

Spring and summer are the natural catabolic times in nature, with the sun pouring energy over us for long, hot hours, energy to be used for activity and evolution. It follows that spring and summer are the ideal times to go on a fast.

Autumn and winter are, in some ways, less suitable times for fasting since this is nature's anabolic phase, when resources are gathered in and stored. The vegetable kingdom withdraws from energy production and concentrates everything on storage and reproduction. Fruits, seed and nuts are formed containing the seeds of a new generation. Energy is withdrawn from leaves and flowers, and put into roots and tubers for storage and use in the next season. The animal kingdom gathers resources, preserves energy and concentrates on the inward life. However, all that storing inevitably leads to some build-up of rubbish, so when the light returns and spring arrives, the time has come for clearing out and making room for new life and growth.

If you decide to have a bodily spring-clean once in a while, here are some hints and tips to help you get the most out of the experience:

1. Find the name and telephone number of a local health professional, experienced in the use of fasts, whom you can contact for further advice, if necessary. (See Useful Addresses, pages 253–255.)

2. Since fasting is all about resting and using every available resource for healing and repair, it is good to find a restful environment where you can get as much rest as you may need during the fast.

3. Prepare yourself mentally for the experience of fasting, and especially for the possibility of a *healing crisis*, which may occur sometime between days four and seven of your fast. Though mildly unpleasant, healing crises are a sign that the healing process is working well, and that the body has plenty of energy to mount a full-scale clean-up operation to remove stored toxins and the debris of old and diseased tissue. All the symptoms result from the higher levels of waste material in the bloodstream produced by the catabolic process and may include:

Mild depression	Vague aches and pains in
Irritability	the joints
Insomnia	Bad taste in the mouth
Weakness	Nausea
Teeth and tongue feeling	Pimples
coated	Increased catarrh
	Diarrhoea

However, the symptoms of a healing crisis produced by a catabolic diet usually disappear within three or four days of their appearance. If you experience symptoms which last longer than this (or which are too severe for comfort), either stop your diet or talk to a registered naturopath, who can help you decide whether to persevere a little longer. (See Useful Addresses, pages 253–255.) Remember, the end result of a healing crisis is more than just a return to health; it is a positive increase in vitality and well-being, which most people feel is worth some minor discomfort. Of course, recovery from all illness involves some degree of healing crisis; catabolic dieting simply accelerates the process and makes tissue healing more efficient and complete.

In a few cases, nausea during a healing crisis is severe enough to lead to vomiting. If this should happen to you, it is important not to become dehydrated; so if it is not possible to keep water down (or if there is diarrhoea at the same time as the vomiting), the diet should be stopped. Very occasionally, people experience mild giddiness or palpitations during healing crises, but these should be relieved by rest and should last no more than twenty-four hours. If they continue, you should consult a registered naturopath.

4. Decide how long your fast is to go on for, and make sure that you have left yourself enough time, both to introduce the change in diet and to return to normal eating afterwards. As a rule of thumb, for every day of actual fasting you should spend one day introducing the change. Thus a seven-day fast should be preceded by seven days of gradual dietary restriction. For example:

Day 1 – cut out stimulants (tea, coffee, chocolate, smoking, alcohol);

Day 2 – cut out sugar (sweets, cakes, fizzy drinks, etc.);

Day 3 – cut out all processed 'convenience' foods;

Day 4 – Cut out meat and fish (if applicable);

Day 5 – Cut out dairy products (if applicable);

Day 6 – Cut out everything except vegetables and fruits;

Day 7 – Eat only fruit.

The return to normal eating should also be done very carefully, and you should spend as many days gently returning to a normal diet as you spent fasting. Begin with fresh fruit, eaten little and often, for example 50–100g every two hours. Introduce easily digestible fruits first, such as orange, grapefruit, melon, kiwi and soft fruits such as peaches, nectarines and fresh apricots.

On the second day, have a breakfast consisting only of fruit, and then eat a salad for lunch and dinner. Use whatever vegetables are in season, but eat only what is easily digestible, for example: lettuce, celery, fennel, endive, cress, parsley, courgette, avocado, grated carrot and beetroot. If you want a snack in between meals, eat fresh fruit only.

On the next day, have fruit for breakfast again, and then some cooked vegetables for dinner or lunch, perhaps with some boiled rice. After this, you can start introducing other foods you normally eat, with dairy products, meats, stimulants (eg. coffee, black tea, chocolate, fizzy drinks) and alcohol being added last (if at all).

5. Remember, fasting is not a test of endurance, it is a time of rest, recovery and repair. However short or long you fast is up to you, but remember that the first one or two days are always the hardest. If you persist, the feelings of hunger will diminish. Remember also that the symptoms of any healing crisis will pass quite quickly, and usually only last two or three days. After a healing crisis, most people experience a wonderful 'high', and have no problems continuing their fast to completion. This return to vigour after a healing crisis is an indication that the body has freed itself of stored toxins. The urine becomes lighter again and loses its strong odour, the tongue clears and the breath becomes fresh.

6. Whilst it is important to rest whenever you feel tired during a fast, it is also good to keep reasonably active. Conserving energy doesn't just mean staying in bed. Gentle walking, cycling, swimming and sunbathing can all be done at a rate that doesn't lead to excessive tiredness.

7. It is important to avoid getting cold during a fast, because getting cold means using energy to become warm again. So choose your environment carefully.

8. The water you drink during a fast should be as pure as possible. Drink little and often, and as much as your thirst dictates. Some people find it more acceptable to include diluted fruit juices (eg. apple or grape) and/or vegetable juices diluted half and half with spring or mineral water. You can drink as much as you like on a fast, but a minimum of eight glasses (ie. 1.5 litres) of fluid should be drunk each day.

9. Since your cells need oxygen for optimal functioning, you should take the opportunity to think about your breathing when you fast. Make it deep, wide and gentle and, if you are not in an environment where the air is pure and full of life, make sure you get as much life out of the air as you can by doing breathing exercises and getting out into the open as much as possible.

10. Light also has an important role to play in health, and is as good for people as it is for plants. In the old health spas, people used to take regular air-baths, which meant stripping off completely and exposing the whole body to the sun and the air for a short time. About ten minutes per day was reckoned to be ideal. If circumstances allow, you might find such a daily bath both enjoyable and invigorating during your fast.

To recap, here is the list of cautions and warnings that should be understood by anyone undertaking a fast:

1. Never undertake a fast in phases of your life where you need to build tissues, such as during pregnancy, breast feeding or during immobilization after operations or accidents. Fasting is also not recommended for those under the age of 18.

2. Never undertake a fast if you are very underweight or have a history of an eating disorder, such as anorexia nervosa or bulimia nervosa.

3. If you are very overweight, do not undertake a stringent fast without the supervision of a registered naturopath (see Useful Addresses, pages 253–255.)

4. If you are on any type of medication, you should not fast without first consulting the practitioner who prescribed it. If he or she is not able to support you, you could consult a registered naturopath.

5. If you are a smoker, avoid smoking while fasting. It may make you feel extremely unwell and it also diminishes the quality of the fast.

6. Alcohol should never be drunk during a fast.

7. Diarrhoea is a common accompaniment to fasting. However, if it is severe and persistent, you should either break the fast or contact a registered naturopath.

8. Nausea and vomiting are also reasonably common reactions during a healing crisis, but vomiting should not go on for more than a day. Break the fast if it does, and contact a registered naturopath for further advice.

9. If you experience giddiness or palpitations, they should go away with rest and, in any case, should last no longer than twenty-four hours. If they do, seek advice from your chosen practitioner.

The end of a fast is a good time to detect any food allergies that you may suffer from. When the digestive system has had a spring-clean, it is much more sensitive, and therefore your reactions to potential allergens may be stronger than normal. By only introducing one type of food at a time as you break the fast, alarm bells will sound loud and clear (eg. nausea, bloating, wind or diarrhoea), if you hit a food or drink that your digestion disagrees with. We suggest you leave any such foods out of your normal diet, because they are an increased burden to your system and use up energy that you could better spend on the rest of your life.

Note: If you are interested in the idea of natural spring-cleaning, but feel that a total fast would be too severe, you can gain similar benefits by substituting one of the catabolic diets from 1 to 5 in the above regime. For example, one traditional variation of the mono-fruit diet goes like this:

Drink grape juice and water, and eat as many grapes as you like for four days; eat nothing, but drink grape juice and water only during the next four days, and then return to eating grapes again for the last four days.

Conclusion

This chapter should encourage you to use catabolic diets as a way of treating acute illness, and to consider the occasional use of fasting as a way of improving your general health. The techniques outlined above have been used safely for centuries to produce sustainable health and well-being. Remember that it is your body and that you are in control. Deep down, we all know what is good for us and, if we do what is good for us, we cannot fail to be healthy.

CHAPTER ELEVEN

GATHERING RESOURCES

In this chapter, we discuss anabolic diets and explain how you can use them to help you recover from chronic Phase 2 illness.

In naturopathic nutrition, the anabolic diet is a wholefood diet designed to increase vitality and provide the strength necessary to recover from chronic Phase 2 illness. It can be used in all circumstances where catabolic dieting would be too challenging – in other words, when resources are low and vitality is weakened. It can be a first step on the road back to health for all those who feel that they have tried everything to cure their chronic condition, but without success.

Anabolic diets often include particular foods and herbs for their specific medicinal actions, and also for their high content of vitamins, minerals, enzymes and immune-stimulating substances. Anabolic dieting has nothing to do with giving yourself a hard time; it is about creating circumstances that make it easy for you to do well and get well.

Anabolic diets – the principles

Chapter Nine looked at how chronic illness is the inevitable consequence of living our lives on the wheel of disease instead of on the wheel of health, and how exhaustion and chronic illness can be the result of repeatedly refusing to give ourselves enough time and space to deal effectively with stress and minor illness.

Chronic illness also occurs when we use medical treatments (both orthodox and complementary) to keep us going from day to day, but neglect the need for proper rest, convalescence and the change in lifestyle often required to produce full recovery. It is the result of using up so much of our internal resources that we have no energy left to heal.

We all seem to have a built-in tendency to over-estimate our capacity to adapt to change, and often believe that our capacity to deal with stress has no limits. This is hardly surprising because, when we consider the relationship between our ability to perform well and the incentives we have to make us perform well, it becomes clear that we have a pre-programmed tendency to try harder when we are under more pressure. The opposite is also true for most people; ie. if we have no incentive to do anything, we don't do anything very well.

The catch is that when incentive or life-pressure causes us to perform well in life, we get rewarded; and when we get rewarded for things, we tend to keep doing them. For example, working late may get us promotion, not having too much time off when we're ill may get us a pay rise, putting extra money into the bank may encourage the bank manager to lend us money to get something we want now, rather than wait; and so on. All this would be fine if it were not for one basic fact: our capacity to respond to increased pressure is not unlimited, even if we do like the rewards that increased performance brings us.

We are a part of nature and follow nature's rules. So it is an inescapable fact that though humans may have a *large* capacity to adapt to change, this capacity is finite. If we over-stretch our personal capacity to perform for over-long, we risk sacrificing our health.

This principle can be seen at work in countless situations. The over-ambitious executive, the over-burdened worker, the over-worked mother, the over-stressed student, the unemployed person struggling to eat and live in a system that seems to neither care nor understand – all are at risk of developing chronic illness. But the reason is the same in all cases: whether we create circumstance by desire or suffer it because of lack of opportunity and resources, if we perform beyond our true capacity without allowing ourselves proper time for recovery, we will eventually suffer illness.

We cannot change the past, but we can change the future simply by acting differently from today onwards. A small change in the position of the tiller on a boat can produce a very significant change of direction.

So, if you are suffering from a chronic Phase 2 illness, or are simply tired out, recovering your health and vitality involves three things:

1. A recognition of the fact that, however things may appear, you are living your life beyond your true capacity to stay healthy.

2. An understanding of the old saying 'if you're in a hole, stop digging', which means being prepared to do whatever it takes to regain your vitality in the short term.

3. A decision to reduce your overall stress level and your overall activity level.

This is not to say that you shouldn't perform to the best of your abilities at all times. However, if you are unwell, exhausted or diseased – in your body, mind, emotions or spirit – you are using more energy than you really have, and will not get well until you get some back. So the reason for going on an anabolic diet when you are suffering chronic illness is very simple: it will give you back the energy you need to start getting well again.

Let us briefly recap the main features of Phase 2 illness:

1. It affects people who have been subjected to a period of physical, mental, emotional and spiritual stress in various combinations and who are constantly tired and run-down, with repeated bouts of minor illness and time off work.

2. It produces diseases that are chronic, with a slow, insidious onset and ill-defined symptoms and signs.

3. The original cause may be in the past, or not very obvious.

4. Treatments tried bring only temporary relief.

Most chronic diseases – both physical and mental – fall into this category, eg. angina, asthma, arthritis, migraine, depression, benign tumours like fibroids, stomach ulcers, inflammatory bowel diseases, fungal infections, eczema and psoriasis.

For all Phase 2 chronic illness, whatever other treatments are used, an anabolic diet is a basic necessity to provide strength for healing. It is made up of foods that are highly nutritious, easily absorbed and easily used by the body. An anabolic diet contains the right amount of protein for tissue growth and repair, and plenty of complex carbohydrates for energy. It is low in fat, but contains the essential fatty acids necessary for health. Refined sugars are avoided because, apart from their low nutritional quality, there is evidence that they may depress the function of the immune system, which needs to be working properly, if healing is to take place.

Practical anabolic dieting

Anabolic dieting is extremely simple. All you do is choose foods that you like from the list on pages 140–141, and then eat as much as you like of them, as often as you like and in any combination that suits your taste.

You do not have to make any special preparations; in fact, you could start straightaway. Just decide on a length of time to follow your diet – and then stick to it; three weeks is a good target to aim for. Don't decide now whether or not to continue longer than this, however. As with any new process, it is good both to have a fixed target (to give the process a chance to work properly) and an escape route (in case the process doesn't suit you).

If, after three weeks of anabolic dieting, you begin to feel some real benefit, it is quite safe to carry on for as long as it takes to establish a substantial improvement in your health. What is more, since anabolic diets are based on personal choice, you can always choose to modify yours as your needs change. The important thing is to concentrate on eating healthy things. If you eat enough healthy food, there will clearly be no room for the unhealthy. In any case, the recommended foods in the following list are not fattening, so it is better for you to eat as much of them as you like, rather than spend weeks restraining yourself, only to binge on 'baddies' when the diet is over.

Throughout your anabolic diet, keep in mind that your objective is to regain sufficient energy to allow yourself to get really well again. So, as well as eating health-giving foods, it is important to be kind to yourself in other ways. Allow as much time as you can for rest, and do your best to avoid things which you find stressful. Proper rest and avoiding stress are parts of your diet, not just additional luxuries. You should also take your time while you eat and, if possible, have a short period of quiet relaxation after each meal. On the other hand, some gentle daily exercise not connected with work (such as walking, swimming, stretching or light gardening) should also be a part of your daily regime.

A few days into your anabolic diet, you may start to experience some mild unwellness, such as headache, 'flu-like symptoms or slight diarrhoea; but don't worry. These are positive signs which suggest that your vitality is returning. The low period will only last a few days, and then your energy levels will start to rise. You will start to feel better in yourself, the feeling of exhaustion will lift and you will notice an overall improvement in your state of health.

However, it is important that you don't use up any new-found energy as soon as it arrives by rushing back too soon to the lifestyle that caused you to become unwell in the first place. Use your vitality for healing. Keep on taking good care of yourself, eating well, avoiding stress and resting as much as possible for several weeks after you first notice signs of actual improvement.

Making a real investment in your own good health at this stage could alter the rest of your life. At best, you will witness a slow, but complete recovery from illness that may have been with you for years. At worst, your increased vitality will significantly enhance the beneficial effects of any treatments you may be undergoing to help you get well.

Recovering from chronic illness is about appreciating your self-healing ability and giving it the credit it deserves for keeping you going, despite difficult circumstances. Respecting your own needs is an acknowledgment of the fact that you can only take care of others, if you take care of yourself first. If you can use your energy for improving your own health, your example will inspire others to do the same.

When a period of anabolic dieting has allowed you to gather strength and has substantially restored your vitality, it can be helpful to use some of your regained energy for a short catabolic diet. As we saw in the previous chapter, catabolic dieting requires a certain level of initial energy to be effective, and so is not generally advisable in chronic illness, unless healing is well established. If you suffer from a chronic disease, it has taken a long time to build up, so it will not disappear overnight. It takes time to overcome the problem by changing the way you live, eat, feel, think and react. You have to concentrate on gathering and conserving your resources and making sure that you use your available energy wisely. However, if anabolic dieting does produce a substantial improvement in your condition, it can be very helpful to complete the period of self-healing with a mild catabolic diet so that you can clear your body of any stored toxins and accumulated waste. See Chapter Ten for further details.

Foods to eat

Here is the list of foods to choose from for an anabolic diet. Eat as many as you like, as often as you like (within reason) and in any combination that suits you. To help you get started, the list is followed by a weekly menu plan, and also some recipes which you may care to try. But remember that the choice is always yours.

Complex carbohydrates Seeds, roots and tubers (eg. rice, pasta, couscous, bulgur, buckwheat, parsnips, celeriac, carrots, potatoes, beetroot, corn).

Protein Beans, peas, grains and green leaves. (Meat is not a good source of protein in an anabolic diet because it is a very concentrated food and may contain residues of hormones, antibiotics, nitrates and other additives.)

Vegetables of all kinds Preferably organically grown, either raw or cooked (boiled, baked or steamed) depending on your taste, the state of your health and your digestion. It may be advisable to start with cooked vegetables if you find raw hard to digest, and then slowly add some raw, if you wish. If you cannot get or cannot afford organic vegetables, use ordinary ones and peel them. In general, organic vegetables contain more nutrients and less water than those produced by intensive farming methods. Just as important, they are not contaminated by sprays and fertilizers which take energy for the body to deal with. Sprayed or not, fresh vegetables are still the healthiest food you can eat because they have not been adulterated by further mechanical or chemical processing.

Fruit Have two pieces per day, either on their own or included in other dishes. Fruit is a very healthy food to eat, but in an anabolic diet the emphasis is on building up energy steadily and not on getting it and using it in short bursts. Most fruits contain simple sugars (disaccharides) which are digested and released into the bloodstream more quickly than the complex sugars (polysaccharides) found in vegetables and grains. So when a lot of simple sugars are consumed, the body has to use more energy to keep the blood sugar stable, thus diverting energy from the healing process. Eat fruits that are in season, and also fruits that improve the digestion, such as papaya, pineapple, banana and grapefruit. Lemons are a good source of vitamin C and don't contain too much sugar.

Drinks During an anabolic diet, the aim is to build up resources, which is done in two ways. Firstly, by eating resource-full foods; secondly, by keeping the digestive workload to a minimum. Drinks should therefore be confined to pure water; vegetable juices (with no added sugar) and herb teas (avoid the artificially flavoured ones as far as possible).

Menu suggestions

On rising
Drink a glass of pure water with the juice of half a lemon, or drink a cup of herb tea (nettle, lemon balm, mint, fennel, rosemary or chamomile).

Breakfast
Choose from the following:

1. Muesli (no added sugar) with soya milk, rice milk or almond milk. Two pieces of fruit.
or

2. Porridge with soya milk, rice milk or almond milk. A piece of fruit.
plus
3. Grated carrot with desiccated coconut, dates, lemon juice and oat cakes.
or
4. Toast and unhydrogenated vegetable margarine with marmite, tahini, nut butter or soya cheese.

Lunch

Eat a large, mixed salad containing a variety of the following and with emphasis on green:

Roots: carrot, beetroot, celeriac, radishes
Leaves: lettuce, watercress, cabbage, mustard, cress
Fruits: tomato, cucumber, avocado, peppers
Stems: celery, fennel
Bulbs: spring onions

Dress the salad with a French dressing consisting of safflower and/or walnut oil, lemon juice, mustard, salt, pepper, herbs (and perhaps garlic).

Add either a baked potato (with vegetable margarine, if preferred – see note below), rice, couscous, hummus, sweetcorn or bread according to your taste.

Dinner

Choose from the following:

Soups: red lentil, asparagus, beetroot, leek and potato, mixed vegetable.

Main: bulgur bake, mushroom pie, couscous, spaghetti with spinach and basil sauce, vegetarian shepherd's pie, vegetarian lasagne, dal with rice, a vegetable paella with rice.

Vegetables: steamed or boiled broccoli, carrots, cauliflower, green beans, curly kale, spring greens, spinach, parsnips, potatoes, sweetcorn, etc.

Recipes for several of the dishes mentioned above are given in Chapter Twelve on pages 149–156.

Drinks

Pure water, herb tea, dandelion or chicory coffee, caro, yannoh (perhaps with soya milk), vegetable juice.

Snacks

Nuts and seeds, bananas, apples, rice cakes, oat cakes, crispbread, raw carrot, celery, fennel or cucumber sticks.

Notes

Spreads Vegetable margarines often contain dairy products and trans fats. Look for 'unhydrogenated' and 'pure vegetable' on the packet.

Labelling Always check food labels to make sure you avoid the following completely:

- Milk (fresh, dried, skimmed), cream, yogurt, butter, cheese, margarine containing milk or milk products (butter, milk powder, whey, casein, caseinate, lactose, milk sugar, lactic acid) and any processed foods containing milk products

- Animal fat

- The following food additives:

E102 tartrazine	E210 to E219 benzoates
E104 quinoline yellow	E220 to E227 sulphites
E107 yellow 2G	E249 to E252 nitrates
E110 sunset yellow	E310 to E312 gallates
E122 carmoisine	E320 butylated hydroxyanisole
E123 amaranth	E321 butylated hydroxytoluene
E124 ponceau 4R	E407 carrageenan
E127 erythrosine	E413 tragacanth
128 red 2G	416 karaya gum
E131 patent blue	E450 di-, tri-, and poly-phosphates
E132 indigo carmine	E466 sodium carboxymethyl cellulose
133 brilliant blue	620 to 623 glutamates, eg. mono-sodium
E142 green S	glutamate
E150 caramels	627 sodium guanylate
E151 black PN	631 inosinate
154 brown FK	924 potassium bromate
155 brown HT	saccharin
E160b annatto	aspartame
E180 pigment rubine	

If you wish to exclude products derived from animals from your diet, you should avoid the following additives (E-numbers):

120, 234, 236, 252, 270, 280, 281, 282, 283, 297, 325, 326, 327, 375, 430, 431, 471, 472, 474, 478, 481, 542, 631, 635, 901, 904.

The following is a list of foods and drinks that you would do well to avoid completely on your anabolic diet:

1. All *sugars* and foods containing added sugar, ie. foods high in simple or refined carbohydrates because they easily upset the blood sugar balance. What is more, research suggests that 100 grams of neat sugar may depress the function of the immune system within thirty minutes of eating it and continue to do so for up to five hours.

2. All *refined* or *processed* foods. Processing upsets the natural balance of food and concentrates certain ingredients out of context. Furthermore, processed foods often contain added sugar, salt, preservatives, colourings and other additives. This makes them harder to digest and increases the body's workload to get rid of unnecessary extras and toxic substances.

3. *Fruit juices.* These contain quite high levels of simple sugars, even if they are no-added-sugar brands.

4. *Stimulants*, such as tea, coffee, alcohol, chocolate, strong spices, fizzy drinks. These make you think you have more energy than you really do, and thus make you use more than is good for you. As a result, eating or drinking stimulants often becomes a habit because the initial 'high' is inevitably followed by a 'down', during which the tendency is to want more stimulants.

5. *Non-prescription drugs and supplements* should be kept to a minimum, because they increase the body's metabolic workload. Confer with a competent practitioner to assess what you really need and what you can easily avoid.

6. *All deep fried foods and fatty foods*, such as fish and chips.

7. *Junk food*, such as burgers and other fast-foods.

8. *Additives* like colorants, preservatives and flavourings, which make food look, smell or taste more attractive and give it a longer shelf-life. For the body, additives mean extra work and the risk of allergy.

9. *Dairy products.* Milk, cheese and eggs are high-fat, high-cholesterol foods which can cause allergies and are increasingly at risk of contamination with additives, such as hormones, antibiotics and teat disinfectants, which upset the natural ecology of our intestines and may produce unexpected adverse reactions.

10. *Meats.* Most meats are high-fat foods and contain trans fats that are known to be harmful to health. Also, much of the meat we buy these days suffers from the effects of factory farming and centralized slaughtering and packing methods. It may contain hormones (such as growth hormone), antibiotics, nitrates and other additives. Extensive use of antibiotics, especially in poultry rearing, has bred resistant bacteria, which pose an increasing problem to the farmers and public health authorities. Modern methods of animal slaughter often compound the risk of food contamination with bacteria that cause food poisoning. If you feel it would be too difficult to do without meat for a while, make sure the meat you eat is fresh, organic and, where possible, locally reared and slaughtered.

11. *Fish*. Modern fish farms for salmon and trout routinely dose the fish with antibiotics and other drugs, which are not necessarily good for human consumption. Wild fish also face increasing levels of water pollution, and any pollutants absorbed into their flesh are passed on to the next link in the food chain – which, if you eat them, is you. These need to be eliminated from the body or stored in bone or fatty tissue, and are therefore an unnecessary drain on energy reserves.

Note: If you suffer from an arthritic condition, an anabolic diet may bring you substantial relief. If it does not, however, you may consider modifying your particular diet to exclude some or all of the following foods (known to make some people's arthritis worse):

Wheat	Acid fruits (oranges, strawberries,
Potatoes	gooseberries, blackcurrants,
Tomatoes	rhubarb)
Peppers	Vinegar (including pickles).
Aubergines	

What about milk and cheese?

The all-purpose anabolic diet described in this chapter is dairy-free, so you can use it (including the menus and recipe suggestions) for all situations in which cow's milk exclusion might prove beneficial.

For example, if you suffer from a catarrhal problem, such as recurrent colds, nasal polyps, sinusitis, chronic middle ear infections or recurrent throat infections, you may experience a dramatic improvement in your condition if you cut milk and milk products out of your diet. Hay fever, asthma, skin conditions (such as eczema and psoriasis), candida infections and arthritic conditions may also benefit substantially from milk exclusion. For, despite its reputation as a natural, health-giving staple food, cow's milk may compromise good health in four ways:

1. Some people (particularly children) are allergic to milk protein and may develop eczema, hay fever or asthma as a result of consuming it.

2. Milk is high in cholesterol, and thus a large intake is associated with an increased risk of heart problems.

3. Milk sugar (lactose) is digested in the stomach by an enzyme called lactase, which humans stop producing from about the age of five. This lack of lactase makes it more difficult for our bodies to deal efficiently with milk products; and there is evidence that cases of recurrent non-specific abdominal pain in children and adolescents may be due to an intolerance to milk sugar.

4. Contamination of milk and milk products with hormones, antibiotics and other agricultural chemical residues may produce unpredictable and unexpected adverse reactions in some people.

It is still not clear, however, why people with catarrhal problems, and the other conditions mentioned above, often experience substantial relief when they start to exclude milk products from their diet. If you go back to first principles though, it is quite obvious that cow's milk was designed to feed calves, not humans. Calves have to develop a digestive system that can ferment and digest grass and, relative to their size, they grow much faster than human babies. Cow's milk therefore has a very different composition from human milk. Amongst other things, it may produce fermentation in the intestines; this produces gas, which calves need for digestion, but which humans find uncomfortable or even painful.

On a milk-free diet, you will still get all the important nutrients you need. Many people have been brought up to believe that if they don't get calcium from their milk, their bones will disintegrate and their teeth will crumble. This issue is discussed in detail in Chapter Eight, but suffice to say here, this is simply not true. A huge number of foods contain just as much calcium as milk (and many contain considerably more) and all the anabolic diets mentioned in this chapter will provide you with ample calcium for your daily needs.

Before deciding whether to cut out milk products from your diet permanently, you have to be sure that doing so will bring you some real benefit. If you stick to your anabolic diet conscientiously for three weeks, one of three things will happen:

1. You will experience withdrawal symptoms for a few days, followed by a mini healing crisis with headache, slight nausea, perhaps some mild diarrhoea. After this, you will feel considerably better and will notice an improvement in your catarrhal condition.

2. You will notice nothing in particular whilst you are off milk, but as soon as you reintroduce it after three weeks, your digestive system will start complaining furiously with wind, abdominal pain and diarrhoea or constipation.

3. You will notice nothing in particular whilst you are off milk, nor when you re-introduce it.

If you experience 1 or 2, it is a strong indication to cut milk and milk products out of your diet altogether.

A diet for all seasons

If you have been diagnosed as having a particular disease, you may be wondering if there are any foods which you should eat or avoid to help you recover more quickly. In Chapter Thirteen, we describe twelve common herbs which can be used in food (and other ways) to enhance the effects of anabolic dieting. In general, however, it is much more useful to provide just one set of dietary guidelines that individuals can adapt to their own circumstances instead of recommending different diets for different diseases. In our years of observing and caring for people suffering varying degrees of chronic illness, we have come to the rather surprising conclusion that diseases don't cause illness. In our experience, the real causes of illness are problems (physical, emotional, mental or spiritual) which put people under stress. If stress continues unrelieved, it uses up self-healing energy – vitality. When the self-healing capacity starts to fail, people become ill. When people become ill, they lose their ability to keep their component parts working properly. When particular component parts (or combinations of parts) stop working properly, we call the results diseases.

Since people work in more or less the same way, it is in fact obvious that we will experience more or less the same symptoms as other people when the same bits go wrong. But instead of trying to understand better what it is that makes us ill in the first place, we have got into a habit of dividing our illnesses into hundreds of different diseases, all based on detailed observation of what has gone wrong *after* it has gone wrong. This, in turn, has led us to concentrate our medical efforts into fighting diseases instead of healing their causes.

To treat disease properly, we need to relieve underlying stress and tiredness, and restore the self-healing capacity. To do this, we need rest and energy, which is the basis of the anabolic diet. Of course, it is important to relieve symptoms, if these in themselves are causing stress and using up energy; but no treatment can produce real healing unless the body, mind, emotions and spirit are given conditions in which they can respond to the treatment.

So, although it is common for food and health books to present different diets for different diseases, this book shifts attention away from disease and treatment, and onto healing and health. Rather than give long lists of foods that are suitable for people who are suffering different conditions, we are suggesting an all-purpose anabolic diet suitable for nearly all cases of chronic illness, a regime which gives you control over what you eat on a day-to-day basis and which encourages you to rest and look after yourself.

CHAPTER TWELVE

A TASTE OF HEALTH

This chapter consists of fourteen delicious recipes that you can use to make healthy eating both interesting and enjoyable.

Some of the dishes in the menu plans in Chapter Eleven may be unfamiliar to you, so here are some recipes for you to try.

Red Lentil Soup

1kg/2lb fresh tomatoes
1 medium onion, chopped
1 clove garlic, chopped
Olive oil for frying
150g/5oz red lentils

Salt and freshly ground pepper, to taste
1 vegetable stock cube dissolved in
    400ml/12fl oz boiling water
1 tbs maple syrup
French bread or poppadums, to serve

Place the tomatoes in a large bowl, cover with freshly boiled water and set aside for a few minutes.

Fry the onion and garlic together gently in olive oil until onion goes soft.

Pour away the water covering the tomatoes and rinse with cold water to cool them down. Take each tomato in turn, make a slit near the top with a sharp knife and peel away the skin. It usually comes away easily in large strips. Blend tomatoes (or chop very finely), and place in a large saucepan.

Rinse the lentils under running water in a sieve (red lentils do not have to be pre-soaked). Add to the tomatoes in the saucepan, together with the vegetable stock, maple syrup, fried onions and garlic. Bring to the boil, stirring continuously; then simmer for forty minutes or until the lentils are soft, stirring occasionally. The lentils absorb a lot of water, so you should add a little cold water from time to time to the simmering mixture to keep the soup at the right consistency.

Remove from the heat, put the lid on the saucepan and leave the soup to stand for ten minutes. Just before serving, return the pan to the heat for a couple of minutes, stirring well and adding salt and pepper to taste, plus a little more water, if necessary. Serve with French bread or poppadums.

Asparagus Soup

1 bunch asparagus	2 potatoes, chopped into cubes
Vegetable stock cube	1 tbs flour
1 litre/2pt water	250ml/8fl oz soya milk (optional)
2 tbs olive oil	Salt and freshly ground pepper, to taste
2 small onions, chopped	Parsley, to garnish
1 carrot, chopped into chunks	Crusty bread, to serve

Cut the tips off the asparagus about 2.5 cm/1 inch from the top and boil in the water until tender (about five minutes). Remove the tips from the water and set aside. Add a vegetable stock cube to the cooking water, stirring until it dissolves, and set aside.

Chop the rest of the asparagus into chunks and stir-fry gently in the oil, together with the onion, carrot, potato and parsley, for about five minutes. Sprinkle the flour over the vegetables and fry for another minute, stirring continuously. Add the stock slowly to the pan, still stirring, and bring to the boil.

Simmer the soup gently for about half an hour. Then transfer to a blender and blend to a smooth, creamy consistency. Return to the pan and bring to boil again. Turn down the heat and add the soya milk, salt, pepper and asparagus heads. Garnish with parsley and serve with crusty bread.

Beetroot Soup

500g/1lb beetroot, in cubes
500ml/1pt water
250ml/½pt orange juice

Salt to taste
2 tsp dill (dried or freshly chopped)

Put the beetroot in a big pot, together with the water. Bring to the boil, simmer partly-covered until the beetroot goes soft (about fifty minutes). Blend the cooked beetroot (together with the cooking water) with all the remaining ingredients until you have a smooth, deep-red coloured soup.

Heat through and serve hot, or put in the fridge to chill and serve cold.

Bulgur Bake

200g/7oz bulgur
1 onion, chopped
250g/8oz tofu, chopped into small
  chunks
250g/8oz mushrooms, sliced
250g/8oz carrots, grated
1 medium courgette, chopped into
  small chunks

500ml/1pt water
1 vegetable stock cube
2 tbs olive oil
1 tsp paprika
2 tsp basil
3 tbs soya sauce
2 tbs lemon juice
Salt and pepper to taste

Put the water in a large saucepan together with the stock cube. Bring to the boil, remove from the heat and add the bulgur. Stir well, cover and set aside.

Heat the oil in a frying pan or wok, add the onion, tofu, mushrooms, paprika and 1 tsp of basil and stir fry for about five minutes. Add the soya sauce, remove from the heat and then transfer the stir-fried ingredients to the saucepan containing the bulgur, together with the courgettes, carrots, lemon juice, salt and pepper.

Stir well and then transfer the whole mixture to an ovenproof dish. Sprinkle with the remaining basil and cook in the middle of a moderate oven (180°C/350°F/gas mark 4) for about 30 minutes. Serve with steamed broccoli.

Mushroom Pie

Olive oil for frying
1 clove garlic, crushed
1 shallot, finely chopped

½kg/1lb mushrooms, chopped into thick
  slices
1 tsp fresh rosemary

I tbs soya sauce

I flat tbs fine cornflour, dissolved in a
little water

Some unsweetened soya milk

Salt and freshly ground pepper, to taste

Enough shortcrust pastry to line and
cover a medium-sized pie tin

New potatoes and carrots, to serve

Heat the oil in a frying pan. Add the garlic and the shallot, and fry gently until soft.

Next, add the mushrooms and continue to cook until the mushrooms start to give out their liquid. Add the rosemary and continue to cook gently for another five minutes.

Add the soya sauce and the cornflour mixture to the pan, together with a splash of soya milk. Bring slowly to the boil, stirring continuously. As the mixture thickens, add some more soya milk until the liquid surrounding the mushrooms is smooth and creamy.

Add salt and pepper to taste, and then transfer the mixture to the pie tin lined with shortcrust pastry. Add a pastry pie lid and then cook in a moderate oven (200°C/400°F/gas mark 6) for twenty to thirty minutes, until the pie crust is a light, golden brown. (Remember to cut a couple of slits in the pie lid before cooking.)

Serve with new potatoes and carrots.

Couscous

2 tbs olive oil

I tsp turmeric

2.5–5 cm (1–2 in) cinnamon stick

½ tsp cayenne pepper

½ tsp black pepper

I tsp coriander

2 bay leaves

2 cloves garlic, chopped

I large onion, chopped

I carrot, sliced in chunks

2 stalks celery, sliced

½ courgette, sliced in chunks

I potato, chopped

250g/½lb mushrooms, sliced

I tbs soya sauce

75g/3oz dried chick-peas or I medium-
sized tin of pre-cooked chick-peas

4 tomatoes (preferably peeled and
chopped) or one tin

Some vegetable stock (plus I glass of
red wine – optional)

Salt and freshly ground pepper, to taste

3 fresh, hot green chillies, chopped

400g/14oz couscous

100ml/4fl oz boiling water

Knob of margarine

If dried chick-peas are used, they should be soaked overnight and boiled in fresh water for about an hour before they are added to the dish.

To make the sauce

Heat the oil in a large saucepan or wok. Add all the spices and fry for one minute. Add garlic and onion, then gradually add the rest of the vegetables. Stir-fry for about five minutes.

Add the soya sauce, fry for another minute, and then add the chick-peas and tomatoes. Heat through and add enough vegetable stock (plus the wine) to cover. Add salt and pepper to taste. Cover and simmer for about twenty minutes.

To make the relish

Chop the chillies finely and simmer in a small casserole for about ten minutes with a cup of liquid taken from the main dish until you have a fairly thick, hot relish. Serve this in a small bowl as an accompaniment to the couscous. Beware, however: chilli relish made in this way can be very hot indeed.

To prepare the couscous grains

The instructions for cooking couscous are usually on the packet, and there are many different methods of preparing it. The simplest way is to place the couscous in a large bowl (together with half a teaspoon of salt) and pour on 100mls/4fl oz of boiling water for every 100g/4oz of couscous. Stir well, cover the bowl and leave to stand for two or three minutes. Then add a knob of margarine and stir well to separate the grains (which should be slightly chewy and not too glutinous).

Cashew Nut Paella

250g/1½lb brown rice	1 red pepper, sliced
4 tbs olive oil	125g/4oz green peas
3 chopped onions	1 tsp marjoram
1 clove garlic, crushed	1 tsp parsley, chopped
2 heaped tsp turmeric	2 tbs cashew nuts
3 tomatoes, skinned and chopped	Juice from ½ small lemon
½ litre/1pt stock	1 tbs soya sauce
2 stalks celery, chopped	Salt and freshly ground pepper

Heat the olive oil and gently stir fry the rice in a large, deep frying pan (or wok or karai) until it turns golden.

Add the onions, garlic and turmeric and stir fry for another few minutes. Then add the tomatoes and stock. Bring to the boil and simmer for fifteen minutes. Add the celery, pepper, nuts and peas. Simmer uncovered until the rice is just cooked, stirring frequently and adding a little more water from time to time, if necessary.

Add the herbs, lemon juice, soya sauce and salt and pepper to taste. Stir well, allow a minute for the mixture to heat through. Serve hot.

Vegetable Lasagne

1 large onion, finely chopped	1 bay leaf
Olive oil for frying	75g/2½oz vegetable margarine
250g/½lb mushrooms, sliced	3 tbs flour
100g/3½oz dried vegetable burger mix	½ litre/1pt of unsweetened soya milk
1 large tin tomatoes	2 tsp French mustard
1 tbs soya sauce	1 tsp Marmite
1 tbs tomato paste	Salt and freshly ground pepper, to taste
1 tsp maple syrup	8–10 oven-ready lasagne sheets
2 tsp herbes de Provence	Mixed green and red lettuce leaves, to serve

Fry the onion gently in olive oil in a deep frying pan. Add the mushrooms and continue frying for a few minutes until soft. Stir in the dry burger mix and continue to fry for a couple more minutes. Then add the tomatoes, soya sauce, tomato paste, maple syrup, herbes de Provence and bay leaf, and mix thoroughly. Bring to the boil and then simmer gently for a few minutes. Adjust the seasoning and then set aside.

Melt the margarine in a saucepan over a moderate heat. Remove from the heat and slowly stir in the flour until you have a yellow paste. Return the pan to a low heat and very gradually stir in half the soya milk, forming a thick cream. Add the mustard and Marmite, stir well and then gradually add the rest of the soya milk, stirring continuously. Check the seasoning (the lasagne topping should taste quite salty in the pan) and continue to heat until the mixture thickens slightly. Set aside.

Take a medium-sized rectangular casserole dish and pour half the tomato and mushroom mixture into the bottom. Spread it out evenly and then cover with a single layer of lasagne sheets (breaking some into pieces, if necessary to cover the whole area). Pour in the remaining tomato and mushroom mixture, spread out evenly and then add a second layer of lasagne sheets. Cover this layer with the lasagne topping sauce and cook in the middle of a moderately hot oven (200°C/400°F/gas mark 6) for about thirty minutes until the lasagne softens and the top goes golden brown.

Serve with a crisp salad of mixed green and red lettuce leaves.

Shepherd's Pie

750g/1½lb potatoes
2 carrots
2 parsnips
1 leek
2 onions
60g/2oz vegetable margarine or 4 tbs oil
Soya milk

30g/1oz dry vegetable burger mix (or
  wholemeal flour)
1 tsp Marmite
60g/2oz hazelnuts, chopped finely
50–100g/2–3oz green peas
Fresh seasonal vegetables, to serve

Clean and chop the potatoes into halves or quarters and boil them in salted water until soft. Drain, keeping the potato water. Meanwhile, clean and chop the vegetables into small chunks. Mash the potatoes with half of the margarine (or oil) and the soya milk. Check and adjust the seasoning and set aside.

Boil the carrots, parsnips and leeks until soft and then drain, adding the water to the potato water, and set aside.

Fry the onions in the rest of the fat or oil. Add the burger mix, stir well and then slowly add 250ml/½pt of the vegetable water and bring to the boil. Add the Marmite, chopped nuts and the green peas. Stir well, check the seasoning and leave to simmer over a low heat for a few minutes.

Grease a medium size ovenproof dish. Pour in the vegetables, then the nut and peas mixture and spread out evenly. Cover with an even layer of mashed potato.

Cook in a moderate oven (180°C/350°F/gas mark 4) for twenty minutes. Just before serving, brown the potato topping under a hot grill. Serve with lightly cooked fresh seasonal vegetables.

Spaghetti with Spinach and Basil Sauce

½kg/1lb fresh spinach leaves
Olive oil for frying
1 clove garlic, crushed
6 leaves fresh basil
1 tbs soya sauce

A dash of lemon juice
2 tbs soya milk
Salt and freshly ground pepper, to taste
1 packet of durum wheat tagliatelle

Cut the ends off the stems of the spinach and place in a large bowl of water to rinse off any dirt.

Put some olive oil in a large pan and gently fry the garlic for one minute.

Drain the spinach leaves and put them into the saucepan on top of the garlic. Put the lid on the pan, turn up the heat a little and wait for the spinach to turn into a soft mass. You should stir the mixture once or twice whilst it is cooking to make sure that the garlic is not sticking to the bottom of the pan.

Transfer the cooked spinach mixture to a blender and add the other ingredients (except the tagliatelle). Blend to a smooth, light cream and adjust the seasoning.

This is a sauce with a taste that is at once strong and delicate. Too little salt and the flavour won't emerge; too much and it will be drowned.

Transfer the sauce back to a saucepan and keep on a very low heat whilst the tagliatelle is cooking in a pan of fiercely boiling salted water with some olive oil in it.

The pasta should be cooked enough to make it easy to chew, but not so much that it loses its bite.

Arrange the cooked tagliatelle in a large serving bowl and pour over the spinach sauce. Grind a little black pepper over it before serving.

This dish goes particularly well with a side dish consisting of mushrooms and onions fried together in a little olive oil or margarine, with a little fresh rosemary. Just before serving, add one or two tablespoons of soya sauce to season the onion and mushroom mixture.

Dal with rice

75g/3oz red lentils, rinsed in cold water	1 tsp turmeric
1 bay leaf	¼–½ teaspoon chilli powder (to taste)
1 small stick cinnamon	¼ tsp salt
1 vegetable stock cube	Small pinch asafoetida (optional)
Olive oil or margarine for frying	2 shallots, chopped small
2 tsp ground cumin	Squeeze lemon juice

Place the lentils in a saucepan with the bay leaf, cinnamon stick and stock cube and cover with water. Bring to the boil, stirring often; then simmer. As the lentils cook, the water will be absorbed, so you will need to go on adding small amounts of water and stirring well as they cook.

Heat the oil or margarine in a frying pan and add the cumin, turmeric, chilli and salt (and asafoetida). After a minute, add the chopped shallots and fry until soft. Add the lemon juice and transfer the contents of the frying pan to the pan containing the simmering lentils. Stir well and continue to cook (stirring occasionally and adding water if necessary) until lentils are very soft. Then turn off the heat, put a lid on the pan and leave the dal to sit for five minutes before serving with rice, on its own or as part of a larger Indian meal.

Winter Salad

250g/½lb red cabbage, finely chopped
2 eating apples, cut in small cubes

75g/2½oz walnuts, chopped
Salad dressing (see below)

Mix the cabbage and apples with the nuts and the dressing (see below).

Serve with French bread as an hors d'oeuvre or as a side dish.

Salad Dressing

Salad dressings are very personal things, so it is not easy to give precise amounts for the various ingredients. Play around with the following method until you produce something that suits your taste.

½ jam jar good olive oil or safflower oil (cold pressed)
2 tbs walnut oil (or another nut or seed oil of your choice)
2 tbs wine vinegar or cider vinegar or lemon juice
2 tsp maple syrup

I tsp fresh or dried herbs (Anything will do. Basil and oregano are particularly good.)
½ tsp salt
Twist freshly ground black pepper
Dash soya sauce

Mix all the ingredients together in a jam jar and shake well until you have an evenly blended dressing.

Try adding half a clove of crushed garlic, or a teaspoon of mild mustard, or a tablespoon of tahini (sesame paste) or even all three to the above.

The trick with salad dressing is not to overdo the sour (vinegar or lemon) taste. If using lemon juice, it is vital to use a lemon that is as ripe as possible. It is best to start by adding only some of the vinegar or lemon, and then slowly add more until you feel that you have a dressing you really like.

Home-made Almond Milk

Per serving
Take a good handful of shelled almonds and place them in a pan of boiling water for two minutes. Drain and then peel/rub off the thin, brown skin with your fingers or the edge of a knife. Put the peeled almonds in a blender with 100ml/3½fl oz cold water. Start the blender and add more water, little by little, until you get an almond milk of a consistency that suits your taste.

Almond milk is delicious poured over muesli and other breakfast cereals. You can add a little maple syrup and a pinch of salt to help bring out the gentle flavour. It can also be sweetened with a little concentrated apple juice, which gives the almond milk a creamy consistency.

CHAPTER THIRTEEN

A SIMPLE FOOD PHARMACY

In this chapter, we describe the use of some common plants in the treatment of illness and give examples of how they can be incorporated into simple, nutritious recipes to enhance your diet.

Plants have been used for their medicinal properties in all the great ancient civilizations, and the experience of people over the ages bears testimony to the health-giving properties of herbs, vegetables and fruits. Although the earth supports many thousands of plant species, the human race makes regular use of just a few hundred, and most people include less than fifty plants in their diet on a regular basis.

This chapter will look at a selection of twelve well-known and easily accessible medicinal plants to show how your food can be your medicine and your medicine can be your food. The information forms a simple self-help food pharmacy, which can help you to deal gently and effectively with many minor ailments. We also hope that it will encourage you to incorporate plants with beneficial properties into your daily meals.

For easy reference, each plant is described in the same way. First, we give the English and the Latin names (as Latin is the international language of botany) and then tell you a little about the history of the plant. This is followed by a brief description of the plant's appearance and habitat, with notes on its general character and its harvest.

We then discuss the plant's medicinal uses, followed by a description of its culinary uses and some tasty recipes to help you turn food into delicious medicines. Finally, there are details of medicinal preparations that can be made from the plant, and any cautions you should observe when using them.

Several of the plants can be used to help the same conditions; this is because – unlike pharmaceutical medicines – they contain several ingredients which have health enhancing properties, not just one active principle. For example, most of the plants chosen have a generally beneficial effect on the digestion, which helps and supports their other, more specific actions.

The best way to get to know about medicinal plants is to use them. If you do, you will soon find those that suit you best. We hope this chapter will encourage you to incorporate nature's gentle healers into your daily life.

Beetroot
LATIN NAME *Beta vulgaris*

HISTORY
Beetroot has been cultivated since the earliest times as a vegetable. It was so treasured by the people of ancient Greece that it was routinely offered – resplendent on a pure silver tray – to the god Apollo in his temple at Delphi.

APPEARANCE
An unmistakeable biennial root vegetable, deep red in colour, with red-veined leaves.

HABITAT
A native of southern Europe, beetroot is derived from the Sea Beet, which grows wild on the coasts of Europe, North Africa and Asia.

CHARACTER
The root is sweet and strong tasting, when raw, but has a more gentle flavour, when cooked. The leaves taste a bit like spinach, for which they can be used as a substitute.

HARVEST
Late summer or early autumn. The leaves can be used throughout the whole of the summer.

MEDICINAL USES
Beetroot is known to herbalists as the vitality plant. The root is rich in vitamins and minerals (especially iron and magnesium) and the leaves are a good source of calcium. In the old English tradition, beetroot was said to be good for the blood, and this is reflected in its modern use in the relief of chronic illness of all sorts, including chronic infections and ME (myalgic encephalomyelitis). An American physician, Professor Koch, claims that beetroot juice is useful in the treatment of hepatitis, nephritis and polio;

many practitioners have also reported encouraging results in cases of cancer, particularly leukaemia. Beetroot is a cheap, non-toxic and widely available supportive, treatment for conditions involving the blood and immune system.

CULINARY USES
Both the leaves and root are edible, boiled or raw.

RECIPES

Beetroot Salad

2 beetroots, cooked and peeled	French dressing (oil, lemon juice, mus-
1 small onion, finely chopped	tard, maple syrup, garlic, salt and
Salt	freshly ground black pepper)
1 endive, chopped	1 bunch of watercress, chopped

Chop the beetroot in ½cm/¼in thick sticks. Put in a salad bowl and mix with onion and a little salt. Add the endive and the dressing. Garnish with watercress.

MEDICINAL PREPARATIONS
Beetroot can be used – raw, juiced, boiled, stewed or baked – as a medicine to improve vitality in all chronic illness. The average dose for an adult is two medium-sized roots per day.

If you have a vegetable juicer, here is a recipe for a blood purifying juice: Take equal amounts of beetroot, carrot, celery, tomato and a lemon, and make a juice of them. Drink one or two wineglasses per day for three weeks.

CAUTIONS
The red pigment in beetroot may colour faeces and urine red, if taken in large amounts. This effect is harmless, however, and disappears as soon as you stop taking the root.

Dandelion
LATIN NAME *Taraxacum officinalis*

HISTORY
The name 'dandelion' came from the French *dente de lion* (teeth of the lion), a reference to the characteristic saw-tooth shape of the leaves. *Taraxacum* comes from the Greek words meaning 'disorder' (*taraxos*) and 'remedy' (*akos*).

The French common name for dandelion is *pis-en-lit*, because the leaves have a strong diuretic action.

The first mention of the dandelion as medicine is in the works of Arabian physicians in the tenth and eleventh centuries. In Britain, the oldest reference is in the writings of the Welsh physicians of Myddfai in the thirteenth century. Since medieval times, dandelion has been used widely as a remedy for liver complaints, and also as a general spring tonic and blood cleanser.

APPEARANCE

The bright yellow flower of the dandelion is so well known as to need no description. Its root is fleshy and brittle, dark on the outside but white on the inside, with a bitter milk-white juice.

HABITAT

Dandelion will grow almost anywhere in the temperate zone, and is a common sight in pastures, meadows, gardens and waste grounds all over Europe and North America. Being one of the first spring flowers, dandelion is very important to bees. The beautiful yellow flower can be seen opening to the sun and closing at night, and in bad weather.

CHARACTER

Herbalists think of dandelion as a bitter, astringent plant.

HARVEST

Young leaves for use in salads should be harvested in early spring, before they go bitter. For drying and tea making, dandelion leaves can be harvested any time. The roots (which should be large, fleshy and well-formed) are best collected in autumn, and should be dug up during wet weather and then hung in a warm, dark, airy place to dry for about a fortnight. Try not to break the roots or cut them before they are dried. Store dried roots in a dry place – preferably in tins – to avoid mould.

MEDICINAL USES

Dandelion leaves are an excellent source of vitamins and minerals, especially vitamin C, beta-carotene, iron and potassium. They are also strongly diuretic and so can be used to relieve water retention caused by heart disease. Dandelion root is a general tonic, with particular actions on the liver and kidneys. It helps the body to eliminate toxic wastes and also acts as a gentle laxative. Dandelion root can be of benefit in all conditions affecting the liver and gall-bladder, and also has a traditional use in the treatment of eczema.

CULINARY USES

The young leaves are delicious eaten raw and are very popular in France, where the crisp and slightly bitter leaves are enjoyed in green salads.

Dandelion leaves are also a tasty addition to pâté sandwiches, sprinkled with salt and a little lemon juice. In France also, the roots are sometimes cooked as a vegetable, as well as being sliced raw and added to salads. Dandelion leaves can be prepared like spinach and used as a side dish.

RECIPES

Dandelion Stir-Fry

2 tbs olive oil
1 clove garlic, crushed
2 small onions, chopped (or shallots)
Pinch of nutmeg
200g/7oz dandelion leaves (approx.)

1 tbs lemon juice
A little water (if necessary)
Salt and freshly ground black pepper, to taste

Heat the oil and fry the garlic, onion and nutmeg for one minute. Add the dandelion leaves, sprinkle with lemon juice, fry for one more minute, then simmer gently for a few minutes, adding a little water, if necessary. Add salt and pepper to taste. Serve as a side dish.

Dandelion Coffee

Dig up some dandelion roots between September and April. Wash them and then place in a warm oven (100–150°C/225–300°F) for several hours until they are completely dry. Put dried roots into a dry, heavy-duty frying pan over a moderate heat, stirring continuously until they go a very dark brown. Grind in a coffee grinder and keep in a sealed container. Brew like coffee.

Note Small birds are very fond of dandelion seeds.

MEDICINAL PREPARATIONS
Dandelion tea is a traditional spring-cleaning remedy made by pouring boiling water onto the leaves (one cup boiling water to one teaspoon dried leaf or two fresh leaves). Leave to infuse for five to ten minutes. Drink one cup in the morning – not in the evening or else you will almost certainly have to get up in the night to use the lavatory!

A **dandelion broth** can be made from the root by slicing and boiling it in water (one teaspoon per cup) for fifteen minutes, straining and drinking one to two cups per day. This improves liver function.

For the **dandelion cure**, soak 50g (2oz) of chopped dandelion root in 200ml (8fl oz) of hot water for one hour. Bring the mixture to the boil for a few minutes, add one teaspoon leaves, and leave to stand off the heat for ten more minutes. Strain and drink one cup of the resulting liquid every morning for three weeks as an aid to digestion and to help remove excess water from the body.

CAUTIONS

Dandelion root should not be used in cases of gastritis, ulcers or irritable colon, and particularly not by anyone suffering from urinary incontinence (unless under the supervision of a competent practitioner).

Because of its diuretic action, it is always best to take this herb in moderate doses, and only in the early part of the day.

Fennel

LATIN NAME *Foeniculum vulgare*

HISTORY

Fennel has been used as a culinary and medicinal herb since ancient times. The Greeks called it *marathron*, from the word *maraiono*, meaning to grow thin. Poor people used to eat fennel seeds to satisfy hunger cravings, and it is still used as a slimming aid.

In medieval times it was used as an ingredient in incense, designed to raise spirits. It was also used to relieve sore eyes and eyelids, and to improve eyesight.

APPEARANCE

A tall, slim plant with winged, feathery leaves and small, yellow flowers. There are several varieties of fennel, all of which have a distinctive sweet licorice fragrance.

The fennel sold by greengrocers as a vegetable is an Italian variety, *Foeniculum dulce*, also called Florentine fennel (or *finocchio* in Italian). This type has a pale green, thickened stem, about 10 to 15 centimetres across, with some feathery leaves at the top.

HABITAT

Fennel grows wild all over Europe, especially in coastal areas around the Mediterranean. It is also cultivated in North America, and produces so many seeds that it easily becomes naturalized wherever it is grown. Fennel should not be sown near dill plants, as the two species may interbreed and, as a result, lose their distinctive, individual tastes. According to tradition, it also should not be grown near tomato plants, since it is thought to inhibit their growth and fruiting.

CHARACTER

Fennel is one of the most relaxing and sweet smelling of all the aromatic herbs. It is also credited with mild oestrogenic properties.

HARVEST

The seeds are harvested when they ripen in the autumn. The leaves and stems can be used fresh from spring onwards.

MEDICINAL USES

Fennel has a calming, soothing effect, particularly on the digestion. It is an excellent remedy for easing wind and relieving colic, and improves the digestion of fat and fatty foods. It can also be used as a diuretic and to relieve inflammation.

From very early times, fennel seed has been credited with the power of increasing the flow of milk in nursing mothers. Since it is such a gentle herb, it can be used freely during pregnancy and breast feeding. Its calming, relaxing and digestive effect is passed via the milk to the baby, and can therefore be helpful in the treatment and prevention of infant colic.

A fennel compress (see below) can also be used to relieve tired, sore or inflamed eyes.

Note that the medicinal actions of fennel when eaten as a vegetable are similar to those of fennel seeds, only milder.

CULINARY USES

Fennel makes a fine tasting, juicy vegetable (rather like celery, but sweeter), which can be eaten raw or steamed.

Young shoots of fennel are delicious when chopped raw in salads and boiled whole, like asparagus. The stems can also be used in soups. Sprigs of fennel can be used instead of parsley as a garnish.

A few fennel seeds bring out the flavour of green pea soup and tomato soup, and can also be sprinkled on mashed potatoes to add interest. A few seeds scattered on pastries and breads before baking give a delicate flavour and aroma.

RECIPES

Finocchio Siciliana (Sicilian Fennel Dish)

3 tbs olive oil
1 red onion, chopped

2 fennel, cut in thick slices (lengthwise)
250ml/8fl oz vegetable stock

Heat the oil in a wok, add the onion and stir fry for one minute. Add the fennel and fry for another two minutes. Then add the vegetable stock and simmer gently until the fennel is tender (about five to ten minutes). Serve hot. This dish goes particularly well with mushrooms and/or cauliflower.

Braised Fennel

2 fennel, chopped
1 tsp fennel seeds
½ litre/1 pt unsweetened soya milk
2 tbs olive oil

2 tbs flour
Salt and freshly ground black pepper, to taste

Simmer the fennel and fennel seeds in the soya milk for about ten minutes (until just tender). Remove from the heat, drain, but keep the liquid. Arrange the fennel in a shallow, oven-proof dish. Heat the oil in a saucepan, then slowly stir in the flour until you have a smooth paste. Still stirring, slowly add the cooking liquid and continue to heat gently until the mixture thickens. Add salt and pepper to taste, pour the sauce over the fennel and cook in the oven at 180°C/350°F/gas mark 4 for ten minutes. Serve as a side dish.

Baked Potato and Fennel Dish

1 tbs olive oil
1 kg/2lb potatoes, cut in quarters
1 fennel, sliced
2 red onions, sliced
6 tomatoes, sliced

1 lemon, sliced
Salt and fresh ground black pepper
1 small bunch parsley, chopped
250 ml/8fl oz vegetable stock

Grease an oven-proof dish with oil. Put the potatoes in the bottom and add the other vegetables in layers, finishing with lemon slices. Sprinkle with salt, pepper and chopped parsley. Add the stock and bake, covered with foil, for fifty minutes at 200°C/400°F/gas mark 6.

MEDICINAL PREPARATIONS
Fennel tea Pour boiling water over the seeds (one teaspoon to a cup of water) and leave to infuse (covered) for five to ten minutes. The tea will be stronger if the seeds are crushed first.

Eye wash To make a soothing eye wash, boil one teaspoon of fennel seeds in two cups of water for ten minutes. Strain and cool before use. Apply (using a standard eye bath) as required, but make a fresh preparation for every application.

Fennel eye compress   Dip a clean flannel, a piece of soft cotton or a piece of clean gauze in the eye-wash liquid. Lie down and put the compress over your eyes. Put another towel on top and keep it there while you relax for about 20 minutes.

CAUTIONS
None

Garlic

LATIN NAME *Allium sativum*

HISTORY

Garlic is a plant so ancient that no one is quite sure of its origins. It was widely used in ancient Egypt where, according to Pliny, it had a semi-divine status (being called upon – along with onion – in the swearing of oaths). It is mentioned in old Muslim legends and in the Bible, and has a long-standing association with religious ritual.

Garlic was also popular with the ancient Greeks and Romans, but even in ancient times the smell was not always appreciated. Apparently, a person who had eaten garlic was not allowed to enter the temples of Cybele.

Garlic has been widely cultivated and used in Europe for hundreds of years, and its strong antiseptic and antibiotic qualities were much valued in the past for the treatment of epidemic infectious diseases, such as plague. It has also been used as a treatment for leprosy and, up to the Second World War, it was successfully applied to war-wounds to prevent septicaemia and gangrene.

Even its reputation for keeping away vampires (by hanging a bunch of garlic over the front door) has a basis in fact. A rare version of the disease porphyria – once relatively common in Central Asia, where garlic grows wild – causes bizarre symptoms which make the sufferer resemble the vampire of legend (pointed teeth, great paleness and a complete intolerance of sunlight). The medicinal properties of garlic could, theoretically, bring relief from some of the unpleasant symptoms of porphyria and may thus form the basis of its vampire repelling reputation. . .

APPEARANCE

Garlic belongs to the same family as onions, leeks, shallots and chives. The bulb consists of several whitish-red cloves enclosed in one white skin. Its leaves resemble the long leaves of leeks. The flowers are small and pale pink in colour.

HABITAT
Garlic is thought to have originated in India or Central Asia (or, some would argue, in Atlantis), but is now cultivated worldwide. Like chamomile and lemon balm, garlic has a generally beneficial effect on other plants grown near it.

CHARACTER
Garlic is pungent and strong smelling. Though many do not like its taste in food, it has always been regarded as an important health-giving plant with strong antiseptic and antibiotic qualities.

HARVEST
This should be carried out when the leaves begin to wither, in the late summer. Garlic is best stored in a dark, dry place.

MEDICINAL USES
Research has shown that eating garlic regularly over a period of time can significantly lower blood pressure, reduce the level of cholesterol in the blood and decrease the tendency of the blood to clot. It is therefore useful in the prevention and treatment of cardiovascular disease.

Garlic is also one of the most effective antibiotic plants available, acting on bacteria, viruses, fungi and parasites. It stimulates the formation of white blood cells and is thus an immune system stimulant.

Over the years, garlic has been used successfully to treat infectious diseases of all kinds, including fungal infections (such as thrush, athlete's foot and ringworm), respiratory infections (such as influenza, tuberculosis, diphtheria and whooping cough) and gut infections (such as dysentery, typhoid and worms). It has even been used to help detoxification in cases of chronic lead poisoning.

Externally it can be used to treat ringworm and infected bites and wounds, and also to draw out insect stings and thorns.

Even with the development of modern antibiotics and a more sophisticated knowledge of the nature of infectious disease, many people still regard garlic as the remedy to be tried first when infection threatens, despite the scepticism of some doctors.

CULINARY USES
Garlic eaten as a regular part of your diet is a tasty way of promoting good health. Use it peeled, crushed, sliced or whole (with a cross cut at one end) to give added flavour to salad dressings, dips, stews, sauces and soups. Some hardy souls even add raw garlic to sandwich fillings.

However, it has to be said that some people have a deep and abiding dislike of the smell and taste of garlic, in all but the smallest amounts. It is certainly a plant that deserves respect, and should not be used in cooking in such a way as to overwhelm the taste and character of the dishes to which it is added.

RECIPES
Garlic can be used to add interest to most savoury dishes by frying it gently with some basil (plus a small pinch of cayenne) in a little olive oil for a minute, and then using this oil to cook the other ingredients of the recipe. Never overheat garlic since this will affect its aroma, flavour and medicinal action.

MEDICINAL PREPARATIONS
Single cloves can be eaten raw in small pieces (perhaps with a little bread and water) as a medicinal preparation, up to one clove a day for adults.

Juice   Take half a teaspoon of juice pressed from some garlic cloves in a little water two or three times a day.

Cough remedy   Soak some crushed garlic in a little maple syrup. Swallow half a teaspoon of the syrup, dissolved in a little water, two or three times a day.

External application   Squeeze the juice from some garlic cloves, dilute in a little water, put on swabs of gauze and apply to the affected area. For areas of broken skin, the solution should be more dilute to avoid causing an excessive burning sensation.

Garlic oil   Crush and mix some cloves of garlic with a good quality oil (eg. olive or almond). Rub some oil on the chest and between shoulder blades at the back to relieve whooping cough.

CAUTIONS
The sulphur content can cause irritation of inflamed tissues. It is therefore best to avoid garlic (or to eat only very small amounts) if you suffer from peptic ulcers or any inflammatory bowel disorder.

Eating parsley together with garlic helps to diminish the intensity of the smell, but doesn't completely remove it.

Ginger

LATIN NAME *Zingiber officinalis*

HISTORY

Ginger, the garlic of the East, is yet another plant with a long history of medicinal and culinary use. It has long been valued as a remedy by the Indian and the Chinese medical traditions (having, amongst other things, a reputation as an aphrodisiac) and was also an ingredient in oriental perfumes. Ginger was popular with the Romans, but only reached England in the ninth century, where it also acquired a reputation as a powerful medicine (Henry VII used it as a remedy to combat the plague).

APPEARANCE

A tropical plant with a characteristic, fibrous underground stem, which is used for culinary and medicinal purposes.

HABITAT

A native of Asia, but widely grown in India, West Africa and Jamaica.

CHARACTER

Hot and spicy, with a characteristic heavy and exotic scent.

MEDICINAL USES

Ginger is used to stimulate the circulation and improve the digestion. A ginger tea will warm up cold hands and feet, ease indigestion and reduce flatulence. Since it causes sweating, it can also be used to cool fevers and to help cleanse the body of accumulated toxins. Chewing a small piece of ginger can be an effective remedy for travel sickness (and morning sickness in pregnancy). Ginger tea massaged into the scalp may help to promote hair growth.

CULINARY USES

Ginger is a fundamental ingredient in both Asian and Indian cookery. Gently sautéed in oil with other herbs and spices before adding the other ingredients, it can be used in curries, chutneys, soups and stews. Freshly grated ginger can be sprinkled over root vegetables to add extra flavour, and is particularly good with artichokes. A little ginger also brings out the flavour of chilled fresh melon.

Whether it is used for its culinary or medicinal properties, ginger should be peeled very thinly because the richest oils and resins are found just under the skin.

MEDICINAL PREPARATIONS

Ginger tea Pour one cup of boiling water on to one teaspoon of the freshly grated or sliced root. Leave to infuse (covered) for five minutes. Drink one cup up to three times a day, as required.

Poultice   Grate some ginger into a bowl of fairly thick, cooked porridge. Mix well and then wrap the porridge/ginger mixture in a clean tea towel. Shape to an appropriate size and place on the affected part (eg. the neck for muscle tension or the shoulder for frozen shoulder). Cover with a towel and a blanket. Leave in place for at least half an hour. A poultice, made in this way, can be used on any part that needs warming. It is not too messy to handle and is very easy to shape and size.

CAUTIONS
Ginger can cause irritation, if accidentally rubbed in the eye, so remember to clean your hands thoroughly after handling it. Strong ginger tea may cause a mild headache, and should be avoided by people with a tendency to migraine.

Horseradish

LATIN NAME *Armoracia rusticana*

HISTORY
The origins of horseradish are obscure, but it is believed to have come from eastern Europe. It was used by many ancient cultures, and is one of the five bitter herbs eaten by Jews at the Feast of the Passover (the others being coriander, horehound, lettuce and nettle). In medieval Europe, horseradish root and leaves were popular as a medicine, and the root later acquired a reputation as a remedy for scurvy.

APPEARANCE
Horseradish is a perennial plant with large, pointed leaves that grow to about 45 centimetres in length. The whole plant grows to a height of one metre (three feet) and produces numerous white flowers during the summer. The root is large, white and woody.

HABITAT
It can be found growing wild in muddy swamps near the Mediterranean coast, but nowadays is more commonly cultivated. Though it needs plenty of water to keep the root fleshy and prefers rich soil, horseradish is a very adaptable plant, easily propagated by root division.

CHARACTER
A peppery, pungent smell with a hot, biting mustard-like taste.

HARVEST
Horseradish is best collected in autumn or spring. The fresh root can be

preserved for weeks (even months) in the fridge, or packed in damp sand and kept in a cool place.

MEDICINAL USES

Horseradish is a powerful natural antibiotic, a strong, circulatory stimulant and a good source of vitamin C. It is also a mild laxative.

Horseradish can be very useful in the treatment of colds, 'flu and other fevers, and may help relieve chronic sinusitis. It is an effective cough remedy (especially when made into a syrup), and also has a reputation for getting rid of worms in children and relieving the symptoms of hay fever.

Horseradish poultice applied to the chest can ease the symptoms of bronchitis, and may also be used to relieve sore joints and muscles in chronic arthritic conditions, and to relieve menstrual pain.

CULINARY USES

Fresh horseradish root – scrubbed, peeled and grated – can be sprinkled on to food as a condiment, and makes an excellent addition to hot and cold sauces.

RECIPES

Almond Horseradish Sauce

2 tbs vegetable oil, safflower, sesame, olive or walnut
30g/1oz flour
½ litre/1pt soya milk
1 tbs maple syrup

2 tbs horseradish, grated
30g/1oz almonds, skinned and chopped
Salt and freshly ground black pepper, to taste

Heat the oil gently in a saucepan. Add the almonds. Add the flour and stir for a couple of minutes. Slowly add the soya milk, stirring continuously. Add the rest of the ingredients. Heat through and serve, poured over steamed vegetables or as a burger sauce.

Cold Horseradish Sauce

3 tbs horseradish, grated
1 tsp paprika
2 tsp maple syrup

1 tsp lemon juice
4 tbs soya milk

Mix the horseradish, paprika, maple syrup and lemon juice in a bowl. Add the soya milk and blend or mix until creamy and smooth. Serve as a salad dressing or poured over fresh vegetables.

Horseradish Relish

Blend some grated horseradish with salt, pepper, maple syrup and lemon juice. Serve as an accompaniment to summer salads.

Hot Horseradish Sauce

Add some grated horseradish to a white bechamel sauce and simmer gently for a minute.

MEDICINAL PREPARATIONS

Horseradish can be used medicinally in a number of different ways:

Raw   Scrape and grate some horseradish root and mix with a little grated apple to soften the taste. Take one teaspoonful per day, washed down with some water.

Horseradish tea   Pour one cup of boiling water over one teaspoon grated or chopped root. Leave to infuse (covered) for five minutes. Drink up to three cups per day.

Poultice   Grate horseradish root into some ready-cooked porridge. Mix well and transfer the mixture to a tea towel. Shape to an appropriate size and put on the affected part. Wrap or cover the area with a towel and a blanket. Leave in place for at least half an hour, but take care that it does not feel too hot. If it does, take it off, let the skin cool a little and put it back on again. At the right temperature, there is a sensation of deep, penetrating warmth that goes deeper, the longer the poultice is left on. Horseradish poultice can be used over any area that needs warming. For example, a small poultice over the sinuses and forehead can relieve chronic sinusitis, and a large poultice can be used to relieve backache and menstrual pain.

Syrup   Pour 30ml/1fl oz of water over 30g/1oz of grated root. Leave to soak in a covered bowl overnight. The next day, take a portion of rosehips or other berries, add an equal weight of sugar, put in a thick saucepan, and bring slowly to the boil. Simmer until you have a thick syrup, remove from the heat and cool. Strain the horseradish from the water and mix the water with the syrup – two parts horseradish water to one part syrup. Take one teaspoonful up to three times a day.

Hayfever remedy   Take one teaspoon of grated horseradish washed down with one glass of water once a day, until you notice a beneficial effect. Then reduce the dose to one teaspoon every two or three days until your symptoms are relieved.

CAUTIONS
Large doses of horseradish preparations should be avoided. Horseradish can depress the action of the thyroid gland, and very large doses can cause kidney problems. Horseradish applied directly to the skin will cause irritation, and the vapour may cause watering eyes. Be careful not to rub your eyes after handling horseradish root, and make sure not to allow any liquid to enter the eyes, when using a horseradish poultice to relieve sinusitis.

Lemon Balm
LATIN NAME *Melissa officinalis*

HISTORY
Melissa is the Greek word for bee, and this sweet-smelling herb does indeed attract bees to the garden. Medieval Arab physicians valued lemon balm greatly for its healing, soothing and calming powers. Its ability to clear the head and sharpen the memory caused some to call it the scholar's herb. Avicenna wrote that 'melissa makes the heart merry', and herbalists over the centuries have used it to strengthen the heart and lift the spirits. Paracelsus was also a Melissa fan, claiming that it had the power to rejuvenate the nervous system.

APPEARANCE
Melissa is a perennial plant that dies down in winter and reappears in the spring. It looks rather like mint, but gives off an unmistakeable scent of lemon when the leaves are touched. The leaves are arranged in pairs on a square stem, and pale rose-pink/white flowers appear in whorls above each pair of leaves.

HABITAT
Melissa is native to southern Europe and the Mediterranean coast, and is especially abundant in mountain regions. It was introduced into British gardens hundreds of years ago, and has since become naturalized in the south of Britain.

Melissa is a plant that likes plenty of space, sunshine, good soil and plentiful water. Many gardeners plant lemon balm amongst vegetables and fruit trees to attract bees and improve pollination.

CHARACTER
Lemon balm – as its name suggests – is a cheerful, sunny, refreshing and soothing herb.

HARVEST
Lemon balm is best used fresh, and can be harvested in small amounts, as required. It is not an easy plant to dry, and dried Melissa loses some of its delicate flavour and beneficial properties.

MEDICINAL USES
Lemon balm is, above all, a gentle herb and an excellent remedy for children. It is cooling, calming and soothing, and can be taken as a tea in cases of fever, coughs and sore throats.

Its gently relaxing effect makes it useful for all conditions of the nervous system, including tension headaches and migraines, and it can be very effective in the relief of insomnia, mild depression and anxiety. Melissa is an important herb in the treatment of high blood pressure, and is also a good digestive remedy in cases of indigestion, wind and colic.

Lemon balm tea, added to a bath, may help ease menstrual pain, and a poultice of crushed leaves will soothe cuts, grazes and insect bites and speed up wound healing.

It is also an important ingredient in 'Carmelite Water', a relaxing, digestive tonic consisting of spirit of lemon balm, lemon peel, nutmeg and angelica root, which was used in olden times to relieve nervous headaches and 'neuralgic affections'.

The volatile oil of lemon balm is widely used in perfumery and aromatherapy.

CULINARY USES
The soft, spicy flavour of lemon balm adds freshness to salads. It is a good addition to cauliflower soup, and is particularly good, when sprinkled on cooked mushrooms.

RECIPES

Bananas with Strawberries

A little plain sesame (or olive) oil or vegetable margarine
4 bananas, peeled and sliced in half lengthwise

4 tbs maple syrup
8–10 lemon balm leaves, finely chopped
20–30 fresh strawberries

Heat the oil in a frying pan. Sauté the bananas lightly on both sides. Add the maple syrup, mix well, then add the lemon balm leaves. Quickly add the fresh strawberries. Heat through and serve at once.

Cooling Summer Drink

Put the juice of half a lemon in a glass, together with several crushed Melissa and mint leaves. Fill the glass half and half with apple juice and fizzy water. Serve immediately.

MEDICINAL PREPARATIONS

Lemon balm tea   Pour boiling water over the fresh or dried herb (one cup per five fresh leaves or per teaspoon dried). Leave to infuse under cover for five to ten minutes. Drink as required.

CAUTIONS
None

Nettle
LATIN NAME *Urtica dioica*

HISTORY
Nettle is one of nature's most versatile plants. It is invaluable, both as a food and a medicine, and can even be used for making clothes. The name 'nettle' has its origins in the words 'net' (Latin) and 'noedl' (Anglo-Saxon) meaning 'sew' and 'needle' respectively, and linen was made from nettles in Scandinavia and Germany until the early 1900s. Hans Christian Andersen's tale, *The Princess and the Eleven Swans* describes how she wove coats for the swans out of nettles. Nettle fibre is similar to hemp or flax, and can be used to produce very fine textiles, as well as the more traditional sail and sack cloth. Nettles have also been used to make paper, starch, sugar, alcohol and protein.

APPEARANCE
Nettle, one of the world's commonest weeds, is instantly recognizable and needs no description.

HABITAT
The common stinging nettle grows throughout temperate Europe and Asia – and in Japan, South Africa, Australia and South America. As a rule, it is found in places where the soil is rich and fertile.

CHARACTER
Nettle is a strong-looking plant with a slightly sweet 'green' taste and smell. It is best known for its sting (the name *Urtica* is derived from a Latin word

meaning 'I burn'), caused by the chemical histamine contained in the little hairs on the stems and leaves. However, when nettles are boiled, the hairs soften, the histamine is dissolved away and the plant becomes edible. An interesting example of nature's balance is that the juice from nettle stems is a good antidote to nettle stings.

HARVEST
Nettles should be harvested on a fine day, in the morning after the sun has dried off the dew. The young tops should be gathered (before they flower) using gloves and scissors. They can be used dried or fresh.

MEDICINAL USES
A useful medicine, a tasty and nutritious vegetable, a valuable animal feed and a source of cloth and dye – nettle deserves a higher status than that of troublesome weed. Nettle tea has been used for centuries as a blood purifier and spring cleanser, and is an excellent aid to convalescence.

Modern herbalists regard it as a circulatory stimulant, a diuretic and a pancreatic stimulant, which lowers blood sugar levels. It is also known to increase milk production during breast feeding. Nettle is therefore used in the management of skin conditions, arthritis, urinary tract problems, oedema and late-onset diabetes. Being rich in iron, it can also be a valuable remedy in cases of anaemia. Cold nettle tea is a useful external remedy for the relief of burns and minor wounds. A piece of cotton wool soaked in cold nettle tea and placed in the nostril for a few minutes is a useful first aid measure for nosebleeds.

CULINARY USES
Nettle has an old and well deserved reputation as a healthy and easily digestible vegetable. Wash the nettle tops well and boil in a little water for about twenty minutes. Then chop finely and use with other vegetables in soups, stews and pasta dishes. As a side dish, pre-cooked nettles are delicious stir fried with leeks, garlic, salt and pepper. They can also be used as a substitute for spinach (but need a little more cooking water). Since nettle juice curdles milk, it is used in the production of vegetarian cheeses.

RECIPES
Scottish Nettle Pudding

I carrier-bagful of young nettle tops, well washed
I leek, sliced

I head of broccoli, chopped
100g/3 oz white rice

Mix all the ingredients together and place in a muslin bag or thin tea towel, and tie well. Boil in well salted water for about twenty minutes (until the vegetables are cooked). Remove from the cloth and serve with a savoury gravy.

MEDICINAL PREPARATIONS

Nettle tea   Pour boiling water on the herb (one teaspoon dried or two fresh tops per cup). Leave to infuse for five to ten minutes then strain. Dose: up to three cups per day.

Hair rinse   Nettle tea can be used as a final rinse to give hair extra shine.

CAUTIONS

Uncooked nettle should always be handled with great respect and never eaten. The hairs on the stems and leaves act like tiny hypodermic needles when broken, injecting their chemical contents under the skin and provoking an uncomfortable allergic reaction.

Parsley

LATIN NAME *Petroselinum crispum (or Petroselinum sativum)*

HISTORY

In Greek mythology, parsley was said to have sprung from the blood of the hero Archemorus, and the ancient Greeks used to crown their victors with parsley garlands. It was also used in funeral rites. Parsley's reputation as a medicinal herb can be traced back as far as the first century AD, and it has been used over the centuries as a diuretic, tonic and digestive remedy.

APPEARANCE

Common parsley is a well-known biennial kitchen-garden herb, producing a mass of characteristically crinkled, deep green leaves. It flowers and produces seeds in its second year. Italian (Hamburg) parsley is a taller, flat-leaved plant, mainly grown for its long, white tap root, which can be eaten as a vegetable (with a taste like a blend of parsley and parsnip). Flat parsley leaves can be used in the same way as other varieties.

HABITAT

The botanist Linnaeus, who is responsible for much of the classification of the plants we use today, stated that Sardinia was the wild habitat of parsley, from where it was brought to Britain in the sixteenth century. Other botanists consider it native to the eastern Mediterranean region.

Parsley needs good soil with lots of nitrogen and a sunny position to flourish. It can take some time to establish itself in a herb garden because of its long germination time of five to eight weeks.

CHARACTER
Parsley has a gentle, rather neutral, but very characteristic taste and smell.

HARVEST
Leaves can be harvested throughout the growing season. Seeds are best collected when ripe, on a dry day towards the end of the second season. Roots should be collected in autumn and early winter.

MEDICINAL USES
Parsley is one of the most widely used of all herbs. It is rich in vitamins A and C, and also in iron, calcium, magnesium and manganese. Parsley is, in fact, a particularly good source of dietary iron, because its vitamin C content helps the iron to be absorbed from the digestive tract.

Parsley leaves and seeds can both be used for their medicinal action, with seeds being the strongest. The effectiveness of both is diminished by drying and age.

As a diuretic, parsley can be used to remove excess water in heart disease, and can also be used to treat problems of the urinary tract. As a digestive remedy, it will ease wind and colic, and assist in the digestion of protein. It can be used to treat anaemia and arthritis, and also to encourage menstruation and to stimulate milk flow. It is a very useful general tonic during convalescence.

CULINARY USES
Parsley mixes well with most other herbs, and is an attractive and tasty garnish for many dishes – especially potatoes. Parsley oil (olive, safflower or walnut oil flavoured with a little parsley, garlic, lemon, salt and pepper) can be sprinkled over food before grilling, to add a special taste.

RECIPES

Parsley and Potato Tart

750g/1½lb potatoes, sliced
a bunch of parsley, finely chopped
100g/3oz plant margarine
100ml/3fl oz soya milk
1 tbs lemon juice
1 clove garlic, crushed
4 tbs tomato paste

2 tsp maple syrup
2 tbs soya sauce
Salt and freshly ground black pepper, to taste
25cm/9in pre-baked flan shell (bought or home made)

Boil the potatoes in salted water until tender. Drain and place in a large mixing bowl, together with the parsley, margarine, soya milk, lemon juice, crushed garlic, tomato paste, maple syrup, soya sauce and black pepper. Mash until you have a smooth paste. Check seasoning. Fill the pastry shell with the mixture and bake in a moderate oven (180°C/350°F/gas mark 4) for about thirty minutes. Garnish with parsley and serve hot with green vegetables or cold with a crisp salad.

MEDICINAL PREPARATIONS
Fresh parsley can be sprinkled on to food or used for its medicinal action in a tea.

Parsley tea   Pour boiling water over two or three fresh sprigs (or one teaspoon of dried herb) and leave to infuse under cover for five minutes. Drink one or two cups per day. For a stronger action, use parsley seeds (one teaspoon to one cup of boiling water).

CAUTIONS
Parsley stimulates the muscles of the uterus to contract, and so strong doses should avoided during pregnancy.

Peppermint
LATIN NAME *Mentha piperita*

HISTORY
Peppermint was cultivated by the ancient Egyptians, and used by Greek and Roman cooks as a flavouring for sauces and wines. It has been valued over the centuries as a soothing and pleasant aid to the digestion, and is mentioned in pharmacopoeias dating back to the thirteenth century. Although it was not used as a medicine in Britain until the eighteenth century, by 1850 it was being cultivated and grown in large amounts.

APPEARANCE
Peppermint – a hybrid of watermint and spearmint – has dark, square, reddish stems and characteristically-pointed leaves. There are many different varieties of mint, but inter-pollination can make them hard to distinguish from each other.

HABITAT
Peppermint grows wild throughout Europe, and is found in moist habitats along stream banks and on waste land. It will grow almost anywhere,

provided there is plenty of water and good drainage. If stinging nettles are planted near mint plants, the aromatic quality of the mint is then greatly enhanced.

CHARACTER
Peppermint is a fragrant, aromatic herb with an uplifting quality.

HARVEST
Harvest when the plant is just about to flower, on a dry, sunny day in the late morning.

MEDICINAL USES
Peppermint is well known for its digestive properties, and can be used to relieve indigestion, wind, colic, nausea and diarrhoea. It has an established reputation in the management of stomach ulcers and can also be of benefit in cases of Crohn's disease and ulcerative colitis.

Peppermint tea is a soothing remedy for colds and 'flu, and inhalations of peppermint oil can relieve catarrh and ease breathing.

Peppermint – particularly peppermint oil – is a powerful antiseptic. Since it also has a local anaesthetic effect, peppermint oil is useful first-aid for toothache.

Crushed fresh peppermint leaves can be applied locally to relieve pain, including headaches. Peppermint baths can be used to relieve rheumatic and muscle pains.

CULINARY USES
Peppermint tea is a good substitute for tea and coffee, and the leaves can be used to add interest to a variety of dishes.

RECIPES

Mint and Raisin Spread

Take one cup of mint leaves and one cup of raisins. Chop finely and mix with a little hot water. Use as a spread or in sandwiches.

Mint, Lemon and Cucumber Salad

Slice some fresh cucumber thinly. Mix some chopped mint leaves with some lemon juice and salt in a bowl. Pour the mint and lemon mixture over the cucumber and serve immediately.

Mint and Beetroot Salad

½ lettuce, chopped
250g/8oz cooked beetroot, peeled and
   sliced

French dressing
1 tbs fresh chopped mint
French bread

Put the lettuce in a salad bowl, add the beetroot and mint, then pour over the dressing and mix well. Serve with French bread.

MEDICINAL PREPARATIONS

Peppermint tea Pour boiling water over the herb (one teaspoon per cup for dried, one or two sprigs per cup for fresh). Leave to infuse under cover for five minutes. Drink as required.

Bath Add a pot of strong peppermint tea to your bath to relieve rheumatic and muscle pains (and also to help relieve itchy skin conditions).

CAUTIONS

If you are using peppermint medicinally or in your diet, and you are taking homeopathic remedies, inform your practitioner. Peppermint may affect the action of homeopathic preparations. Peppermint oil inhalations should not be used over prolonged periods.

Rosemary

LATIN NAME *Rosmarinus officinalis*

HISTORY

Rosemary is a herb of legend. In prehistoric times, it was dedicated to the goddess of love. The Romans decorated their house gods with it, and it has been used in religious ceremonies for thousands of years. Christians use rosemary in Christening water and in Spain, it is revered as one of the herbs that gave shelter to the Virgin Mary on the flight to Egypt. In many places, rosemary has been used as a safeguard against evil. It symbolizes faithfulness and remembrance, and is used at weddings as well as funerals.

Its tonic, stimulant and astringent qualities were much favoured by the Welsh physicians of Myddfai, who also recommended bath water scented with rosemary to preserve youth and good looks.

Gypsies treasure rosemary above all other herbs, for its beneficial effects on skin and hair. Rosemary also used to be burned as incense in French hospitals, to purify the air.

APPEARANCE
An evergreen shrub, with leaves like pine needles and light blue flowers.

HABITAT
A native to the shores of the Mediterranean, rosemary likes dry and sunny conditions and may live to a great age – thirty years or more.

CHARACTER
Pleasantly fragrant, strong and distinctive, with a pine-like, highly aromatic quality, rosemary is a herb of friendship and remembrance.

HARVEST
Any time during the summer.

MEDICINAL USES
Since ancient times, rosemary has had a reputation for strengthening the memory and focusing the mind. It is said to 'make thee light and merrie', and is a useful remedy for headache and for mild depression. Rosemary is also a good general tonic during convalescence.

As a circulatory stimulant, rosemary can be useful in conditions caused by poor circulation. As a digestive remedy, it can be used to relieve indigestion and wind.

Externally, rosemary can be used to prevent and reduce hair loss, and rosemary massage oil relieves muscle and joint pain. Rosemary oil is also a common ingredient in soaps, shampoos, tonics, oils, perfumes and toilet waters. It is a major ingredient in eau de cologne.

CULINARY USES
Rosemary can be used in any vegetable dish – particularly those with a Greek theme – and it goes particularly well with mushrooms. To blend the taste of rosemary gently into a dish, start by frying finely chopped rosemary together with some onion, before adding the other ingredients.

RECIPES

Spaghetti with Herb Sauce

2 tbs olive oil
1 clove garlic, crushed
2 onions, chopped
2 stalks celery, sliced
4 sprigs of parsley, chopped
2–4 sprigs of rosemary, chopped
6 tomatoes, quartered

1 tbs soya sauce
Juice from ½ lemon
Salt and freshly ground black pepper, to taste
Enough spaghetti for 4, cooked and drained

Heat the oil in a wok. Sauté the garlic and onions together for one minute. Add the celery, parsley and rosemary and cook over a low heat for one minute. Then add the tomatoes and soya sauce. Simmer gently until the tomatoes go soft. Add the lemon juice, and salt and pepper to taste. Put the hot spaghetti in a big serving dish, pour the sauce over and serve (perhaps with some French bread).

Rosemary Soup

2 tbs olive oil

3 medium onions, chopped

1 medium tin chick-peas (or 100g/3oz
    dried chick-peas, soaked overnight,
    rinsed and pre-boiled for one hour)

2 tbs lemon juice

5 sprigs fresh rosemary (or 3 tsp dried)

1.5 litre/3pts vegetable stock

2 tbs soya sauce

Salt and pepper, to taste

Pitta bread, to serve

Heat the oil in a large saucepan and gently sauté the onion and drained chick-peas for a few minutes. Add the stock and the rosemary, bring to the boil and simmer (covered) until the chick-peas are very tender (about half an hour). Add the soya sauce, lemon juice and salt and pepper to taste. Serve the soup as it is, or blend and reheat. Serve with warm pitta bread.

MEDICINAL PREPARATIONS

Rosemary tea Pour boiling water on the herb (one teaspoon of rosemary per cup of boiling water) and leave to infuse (covered) for five to ten minutes. Dose: one or two cups a day.

Rosemary bath Take two tablespoons dried herb or six fresh sprigs, put them in a teapot and fill with boiling water. Infuse for ten to fifteen minutes and then add to the bath water. A rosemary bath, taken in the morning, will invigorate your mind, stimulate circulation and tone up your skin.

Incense An oil burner, filled with water and a few drops of essential oil of rosemary, will quickly and efficiently cleanse smoky or polluted air. A few dried sprigs, burnt in an earthenware bowl, will purify the atmosphere in a sickroom.

Rosemary oil Fill a glass jar with rosemary sprigs, then pour a good vegetable oil over them until the jar is full. Put on a tightly fitting lid and leave the jar on a sunny windowsill for two weeks. After two weeks, filter the rosemary oil into a clean bottle. This oil can be used for massage and will relieve sore joints, aching muscles and tension headaches.

Tonic hair rinse   Put a handful of rosemary in a small bowl or teapot and add a large cup of boiling water. Cover, and leave for at least an hour. Use after shampooing, as a hair rinse.

CAUTIONS
Large amounts of rosemary taken internally can be poisonous, but the herb is perfectly safe, when used in normal culinary or medicinal amounts. The essential oil should not be used externally or internally during pregnancy.

Thyme
LATIN NAME *Thymus vulgaris*

HISTORY
Thyme was used by the ancient Egyptians and by the Romans in the embalming of dead bodies. The name is derived from the Greek word *thumus* meaning *courage* and also *to cleanse* or *fumigate*. Thyme is associated in legend with courage, grace, energy and the devotion of motherhood.

APPEARANCE
A low-growing perennial herb with small, oval leaves and reddish-purple coloured flowers.

HABITAT
Thyme grows wild in Mediterranean areas, but is cultivated all over the world. It was introduced to Britain by the Romans. Its natural habitat is moorland and mountain slopes.

CHARACTER
Thyme is fragrant and pleasantly aromatic. It is warming and sweet, with a sharp and attractive scent.

HARVEST
Preferably between June and August, in the late morning on a dry day.

MEDICINAL USES
All the many varieties of thyme are edible and valuable medicinally. However, two types are mainly used:

1. Common or garden thyme (*Thymus vulgaris*) and
2. Wild or mountain thyme (*Thymus serpyllum*).

Garden thyme is an 'improved' version of wild thyme.

Thyme is a powerful antiseptic and a fine natural antibiotic, which can be used internally and externally. It can be used to treat colds, 'flu, tonsillitis and all kinds of respiratory infection. Thyme is useful in cases of cystitis and urethritis and will also relieve gut infections and infestations (including ascaris and hookworm). Since it relaxes internal muscle spasm, it can be a very helpful remedy for asthma and an effective way of relieving the occasional bout of diarrhoea. It is also an excellent mouthwash for gum disease and can be used externally on cuts and wounds to prevent infection.

The aroma of thyme is long lasting and so thyme can be used to fumigate rooms with a bad smell or atmosphere. A small linen bag of dried thyme can be laid with clothes and linen to give a fresh scent and to keep away insects. Oil of thyme is used in soaps, cosmetics and perfume.

CULINARY USES
Thyme can be used to add flavour and interest to tomato soup and other tomato dishes. It also goes well with olives, mushrooms, courgettes and aubergines.

RECIPES

Mushroom and Thyme Sauce

250g/½lb mushrooms
2 tbs flour
200ml/8fl oz vegetable stock
1 tbs soya sauce
150ml/6fl oz soya milk

1 tsp thyme
Salt, freshly ground black pepper and a
   little yeast extract, to taste
Olive oil

Clean the mushrooms and let them dry. Slice and sauté them in a little olive oil for approximately five minutes. Sprinkle the flour over the mushrooms, stir in well and then add the vegetable stock slowly, stirring continuously. Bring to boil, add the rest of the ingredients except the soya milk and simmer gently for another five minutes, stirring occasionally. Finally, add the soya milk, heat through and adjust seasoning. Be careful not to let the sauce boil too much once you have added the soya milk or it may curdle.

MEDICINAL PREPARATIONS

Thyme tea Pour boiling water on the herb (one teaspoon of fresh or dried herb per cup of water) and leave covered for five to ten minutes. Strain.

Drink in small quantities spread over the day (up to a maximum of three cups per day total).

Mouthwash Make two cups of thyme tea. Leave to cool. Strain and use morning and evening after brushing teeth.

Bath Two to four cups of tea added to bath water can be used to ease rheumatic pains and to relieve skin conditions.

Wrap Soak a piece of linen or gauze (or a clean tea towel) in thyme tea and put it on the skin over the affected area. Put a towel on top and leave for twenty minutes.

Inhalation Fill a saucepan with water, bring to the boil and add two table-spoons of thyme. Put the lid on, turn off the heat and leave to infuse (and cool) for about five minutes.

Put two chairs facing each other. Place the pan on one and yourself on the other. Put a big towel over your head and wrap yourself in a big blanket. Take the lid off the pan and inhale the steam for about ten or fifteen minutes. This has a clearing and cleansing effect on the head, the sinuses and the airways.

CAUTIONS
Thyme should not be used in cases of kidney disease or damage without qualified supervision.

CHAPTER FOURTEEN

FOOD FOR A FUTURE

In this final chapter, we consider the effects of modern food production and distribution methods on the health of individuals, society and the planet, and offer some thoughts for the future.

As the twentieth century draws to a close, food production and distribution systems in the West appear to be coming under increasing strain. Cattle and other farm animals are dying of BSE (mad-cow disease); dairy products are contaminated by salmonella and listeria; crops are routinely covered with pesticides and other poisons; water supplies are polluted by agrochemical residues and by ammonia waste from factory farms.

Monocrop farming methods are damaging soil and wildlife; the landscape is scarred by acres of hedge-less, treeless prairie; farmers are sick from using organo-phosphates and find themselves under constant, sometimes intolerable, financial strain. Cattle, sheep, pigs and poultry are transported in inhumane ways and there is huge expenditure on international food transport systems, which further pollute our already polluted air.

Processed foods contain additives of questionable safety; food is irradiated, sometimes without consumer knowledge; mechanically recovered meat slurry is added to foodstuffs to increase profit; processed food costs are kept artificially low by government subsidy, and supermarkets are driving small food retailers out of business.

Millions of pounds are spent each year persuading us to eat sugar and fat (and drink alcohol) dressed up in pretty packages, with additives to give taste and colour. People have become stimulant junkies – caffeine-containing beverages are world best sellers – and children are hooked on fast foods, sugar and fat. Food supplement companies are following the example of drug companies in their sales and marketing techniques, and baby-milk formulae are threatening the lives of children in the Third World. Third World food producers are exploited by First World food profiteering and, to keep prices up, tax payers' money is being used to trash millions of tons of food in the West while millions starve in the South.

Consider what would happen, however, if we were all to start eating more fresh, organic, locally grown, minimally packaged plant-based foods – supplemented according to taste with some fresh, organic, locally produced, animal-based foods.

The land would be healthier. Farmers would be healthier. Wildlife would be healthier. We would be healthier. Trees and hedgerows would reappear in the landscape. Real markets would reappear in towns and villages. The number of heavy lorries on our roads would decrease. Land, the water supply and the air would be less polluted. Communities in the Third World could start reclaiming their land to produce primary plant foods for their own consumption, and householders in urban inner cities could even start to use the derelict wastelands around tower blocks and housing estates to grow fresh fruit and vegetables.

In short, there would be a revolution. We would have changed the world by changing what we put in our mouths.

Throughout this book, we have stressed the importance of following nature's example as a way of promoting health, but if we in the West are to return to a more natural way of eating, we need to start looking at food in a new way.

If you studied biology at school, you probably came across the concept of the food chain. As usually described, the humble plant is at the bottom of this chain. Plants are eaten by gentle herbivores, who in turn are eaten by the stronger carnivores. Man, with his intelligence and his weapons, is placed at the head of the food chain, since he has the power to kill and eat all other species on the earth, should he so desire.

But what if, instead of assuming that the strongest should come first, we reconstructed the food chain, putting those species most useful to nature *as a whole* at the top, and those least useful at the bottom? In such a 'life chain', the plants would be at the top because they turn the sun's energy into food for the rest of creation and help to ensure the quality of the soil, the air and the water. Then would come the fruit, nut and seed eaters who, rather than cause a net loss of life by their eating habits, help to spread plant species around the environment and return nutrients back to the soil with their manure. Some also provide food for creatures below them on the chain.

Next would come the grazing herbivores, whose wastes return nourishment to the land and who provide food of many different types for other species, usually by losing their own lives. Then would come the pure carnivores, playing a part in maintaining the overall balance of nature and, in the end, providing food for the scavengers.

And at the bottom of the chain, strangely isolated, would come man, using his awesome power to take whatever he chooses from the world around him but, on the whole, only stopping to give something back when his immediate interests are threatened. *Homo sapiens* is the only species on earth that takes from nature more than it really needs for its survival. Instead of returning waste to the soil, man creates toxic, sometimes un-degradable rubbish, with which he pollutes the land, the rivers, the seas and the air. Thinking that he is at the top of the food chain, man is upsetting the balance of nature and even risks destroying himself.

Of course, human kind also has another nature – one of tenderness, kindness and compassion. We have the intelligence to climb the stairway to heaven and beyond, as well as the wherewithal to create a living hell. We have an infinite capacity for love despite a tendency to get side-tracked by our wants and desires. Our greatest gift is our capacity for choice and, despite the commonly held belief, for us in the West choice is real and ever present. We can choose to stop taking more than we actually need from the earth; to live simply and therefore make it possible for others simply to live.

And we can do this without becoming religious or fanatical or political, simply by starting to change our diet in a way that both benefits our health, the health of our fellow humans and the rest of this planet of miracles.

We can start by realizing that we are what we eat.

APPENDICES: FOOD FACTS

APPENDIX ONE

THE NUTRITIONAL CONTENT OF HEALTHY FOODS

The following tables will provide you with a unique and comprehensive nutritional reference source. Used in conjunction with Appendices Two and Three, they will enable you to assess the nutritional value of particular foods in your diet, and will help you to deepen your understanding of naturopathic nutrition.

The tables list the average protein, fat, carbohydrate, fibre, calorie, vitamin and mineral contents of nearly all types of plant food, arranged according to which parts of plants they come from. Any food with an overall nutrient content very different from the group average is listed separately. Foods particularly high or low in just one or two nutrients are referred to in **Notes**.

The average protein, fat and carbohydrate contents of each food group are listed in two ways. First in the conventional 'grams per 100 grams' format, and then as a percentage of the total energy (calorie) content. For example, foods in Group 1a (beetroot, carrot, celeriac, parsnip, swede and turnip) contain an average of 1.1 grams of protein per 100 grams, which means that thirteen percent of their calories come from protein. Potatoes (Group 1b) contain an average 17.6 grams of carbohydrate per 100 grams, which means that eighty-eight percent of their calories come from carbohydrates.

The total fat content of each food group is analysed to show you what percentage of the fat comes from saturated (SFA), mono-unsaturated (MUFA) and polyunsaturated (PUFA) fatty acids.

The energy (calorie) content of each group is given both in terms of kilocalories per 100 grams and in terms of kilocalories per average portion.

The average vitamin and mineral contents of the various plant food groups are listed in separate tables, with foods particularly high or low in any vitamin or mineral being commented on in **Notes**. Average vitamin B12 contents are not included, since these are still a subject of debate (see Chapter Eight). Appendices Two and Three give further details about vitamins and minerals.

The tables in this appendix do not include information on animal-based or processed food products, because they are intended to help you find ways of increasing your intake of health-giving, plant-based foods. Conventional nutritional literature often devotes little space to the nutritional content of plants, so many people are unaware of the health-giving potential of cheap, widely available vegetables, fruits, nuts, pulses and grains.

NUTRITIONAL CONTENTS OF PLANT FOODS

Table 1. Protein, Fat, Carbohydrate, Fibre and Energy

Food	Protein grams[1]	%[2]	Total fat grams[1]	%[2]	Fatty acids as % of total fat sfa[3]	mufa[3]	pufa[3]	Carbohydrate grams[1]	%[2]	Fibre grams[1]	Energy (kilocalories) per 100g	per portion
1. Roots and Tubers												
1a. Beetroot, carrots, celeriac, parsnips, swedes, turnips – average	1.1	13	0.4	12	17	27	46	6.6	75	3.2	33	20
1b. Potatoes – average	1.8	10	0.2	2	23	3	74	17.6	88	1.4	75	135
Sweet potatoes	1.6	6	0.4	3	47	8	41	27.9	91	3.0	115	150
Yams	2.1	6	0.4	2	n[4]	n	n	37.5	92	4.9	153	199
1c. Fresh ginger	1.4	15	0.6	14	n	n	n	7.2	71	n	38	n
1d. Horseradish	4.5	29	0.3	4	n	n	n	11.0	67	7.5	62	6
1e. Radishes	0.7	24	0.2	16	n	n	n	1.9	60	0.9	12	1

Notes: *Beetroot is lower than the average in fat.*

Food	Protein grams[1]	%[2]	Total fat grams[1]	%[2]	sfa[3]	mufa[3]	pufa[3]	Carbohydrate grams[1]	%[2]	Fibre grams[1]	Energy per 100g	per portion
2. Bulbs												
2a. Onions, shallots, spring onions, leeks – average	1.3	19	0.2	7	n	n	n	5.7	74	2.2	28	17
2b. Garlic	7.9	32	0.6	6	n	n	n	16.3	62	4.1	98	10

Notes: *Leeks are higher than the average in fat, spring onions lower.*

Food	Protein grams[1]	%[2]	Total fat grams[1]	%[2]	sfa[3]	mufa[3]	pufa[3]	Carbohydrate grams[1]	%[2]	Fibre grams[1]	Energy per 100g	per portion
3. Stems												
3a. Celery and fennel – average	0.7	28	0.2	19	n	n	n	1.4	53	2.2	10	5

1 Grams per hundred grams of food.
2 Percentage of total energy.
3 sfa = saturated fatty acid, mufa = monounsaturated fatty acid, pufa = polyunsaturated fatty acid.
4 n = figures not available.

Table 1. Protein, Fat, Carbohydrate, Fibre and Energy

Food	Protein grams[1]	Protein %[2]	Total fat grams[1]	Total fat %[2]	Fatty acids as % of total fat sfa[3]	mufa[3]	pufa[3]	Carbohydrate grams[1]	Carbohydrate %[2]	Fibre grams[1]	Energy (kilocalories) per 100g	per portion
4. Leaves												
4a. Greens – brussels sprouts, cabbage, curly kale, endive, spinach, spring greens – average	2.7	38	0.9	28	14	8	60	2.6	34	3.7	29	26
4b. Salads (all lettuces) – average	0.8	23	0.5	32	n[4]	n	n	1.7	45	1.3	14	7
4c. Cress (mustard, cress, watercress) – average	2.3	52	0.8	40	30	10	40	0.4	8	3.2	18	1
4d. Herbs (basil, chives, coriander, dill, mint, oregano, parsley, rosemary, sage, tarragon, thyme) – average	2.6	21	1.6	30	n	n	n	6.4	49	n	49	0.5
Notes: Compared with the average, dill is lower in carbohydrate; rosemary is lower in protein; sage is higher in energy.												
5. Flowers												
5a. Artichoke, green broccoli, purple broccoli, cauliflower – average	3.5	48	0.7	22	22	9	55	2.3	30	2.6	29	15

1 Grams per hundred grams of food.
2 Percentage of total energy.
3 sfa = saturated fatty acid, mufa = monounsaturated fatty acid, pufa = polyunsaturated fatty acid.
4 n = figures not available.

Table I. Protein, Fat, Carbohydrate, Fibre and Energy

Food	Protein grams[1]	%[2]	Total fat grams[1]	%[2]	Fatty acids as % of total fat sfa[3]	mufa[3]	pufa[3]	Carbohydrate grams[1]	%[2]	Fibre grams[1]	Energy (kilocalories) per 100g	per portion
6. Seeds												
6a. Pulses												
Fresh pulses (broad beans, green beans, runner beans, mange tout, sugar snap and ordinary peas) – average	3.9	37	0.6	12	15	12	48	5.7	51	3.2	42	38
Mung beans sprouts	2.9	37	0.5	15	n[4]	n	n	4.0	48	5.6	31	6
Alfalfa sprouts	4.0	67	0.7	26	n	n	n	0.4	7	1.7	24	5
Dried pulses (aduki, black gram, black-eye, haricot, mung, pinto, red kidney and butterbeans, chick-peas, dal, split and pigeon peas) – average	8.1	30	0.5	5	21	10	47	18.8	65	5.5	109	98
Green & brown lentils – average	8.8	34	0.7	6	11	16	42	16.9	60	3.8	105	95
Red lentils	7.6	30	0.4	4	15	15	38	17.5	66	3.3	100	90
Soya products (incl. soya beans, tempeh and tofu) – average	14.3	45	6.0	41	12	19	48	5.8	14	5.1	154	139
Soya flour	36.8	33	23.5	47	n	n	n	23.5	20	10.7	447	89
Soya milk (unsweetened)	4.0	40	2.5	46	12	19	48	1.5	14	n	40	40
Baked beans	4.8	23	0.6	7	21	12	63	15.1	70	6.6	81	109
Hummus	7.6	16	12.6	61	n	n	n	11.6	23	3.2	187	94

Notes: Tofu is lower than the average in carbohydrate and fibre.

1 Grams per hundred grams of food.
2 Percentage of total energy.
3 sfa = saturated fatty acid, mufa = monounsaturated fatty acid, pufa = polyunsaturated fatty acid.
4 n = figures not available.

Table 1. Protein, Fat, Carbohydrate, Fibre and Energy

Food	Protein grams[1]	% [2]	Total fat grams[1]	% [2]	Fatty acids as % of total fat sfa[3]	mufa[3]	pufa[3]	Carbohydrate grams[1]	% [2]	Fibre grams[1]	Energy (kilocalories) per 100g	per portion
6b. Grains												
Wholegrains and flours (barley, buck-wheat, bulgur, couscous, millet, rye, wheat) – average	9.2	11	1.8	5	n[4]			74.0	84	8.2	337	67
Rice products (brown rice, white rice, basmati) – average	6.9	8	1.4	4	n	n	n	82.6	88	3.0	359	539
Rice flour	6.4	7	0.8	2	n	n	n	80.1	82	2.0	366	73
Breads (brown, white, wholemeal, rye) – average	8.8	15	2.5	10	n	n	n	46.8	75	5.9	233	70
Pasta (spaghetti, macaroni, tagliatelle, etc.) – average	12.3	15	2.0	5	n	n	n	72.7	80	5.0	340	782

Notes: *Wholemeal spagetti is higher in fibre.*

Food	Protein grams[1]	% [2]	Total fat grams[1]	% [2]	sfa[3]	mufa[3]	pufa[3]	Carbohydrate grams[1]	% [2]	Fibre grams[1]	Energy per 100g	per portion
Breakfast cereals (muesli)	10.5	11	8.1	20	n	n	n	67.1	69	11.1	366	183
Porridge	1.5	12	1.1	20	n	n	n	9.0	68	0.8	49	98

Notes: *These figures apply to muesli and porridge with no added sugar, and porridge made with water.*

Food	Protein grams[1]	% [2]	Total fat grams[1]	% [2]	sfa[3]	mufa[3]	pufa[3]	Carbohydrate grams[1]	% [2]	Fibre grams[1]	Energy per 100g	per portion
Wheat bran	14.1	27	5.5	24	n	n	n	26.8	49	39.6	206	14
Cornflour	0.6	1	0.7	2	n	n	n	92.0	97	0.1	354	71
Corn-on-the-cob	2.0	15	1.0	17	11	28	39	9.9	68	1.9	54	68
Oatmeal	12.4	12	8.7	20	n	n	n	72.8	68	6.3	401	60
Oatcakes	10.8	10	18.3	37	n	n	n	63.2	53	5.5	445	45
Sago	0.2	–	0.2	1	n	n	n	94.0	99	0.5	355	n
Semolina	10.7	12	1.8	5	n	n	n	77.5	83	3.6	350	n
Wheatgerm	26.7	35	9.2	27	n	n	n	44.7	56	15.6	302	15

1 Grams per hundred grams of food.
2 Percentage of total energy.
3 sfa = saturated fatty acid, mufa = monounsaturated fatty acid, pufa = polyunsaturated fatty acid.
4 n = figures not available.

Table 1. Protein, Fat, Carbohydrate, Fibre and Energy

Food	Protein grams[1]	% [2]	Total fat grams[1]	% [2]	Fatty acids as % of total fat sfa[3]	mufa[3]	pufa[3]	Carbohydrate grams[1]	% [2]	Fibre grams[1]	Energy (kilocalories) per 100g	per portion
6c. Spices (anise, caraway, celery, coriander, cumin, dill, fennel, mustard seeds) – average	17.8	n[4]	18.8	n	n	n	n	n	n	n	n	n
6d. Nuts and seeds (almonds, brazils, cashews, hazels, pecans and walnuts, pine kernels, pumpkin, sesame and sunflower seeds) – average	17.5	11	58.2	84	13	39	41	8.6	5	6.6	627	94

Notes: Hazelnuts are higher than average in monounsaturated fatty acids (mufa).

7. Fruits

Food	Protein grams[1]	% [2]	Total fat grams[1]	% [2]	sfa[3]	mufa[3]	pufa[3]	Carbohydrate grams[1]	% [2]	Fibre grams[1]	Energy per 100g	per portion
7a. Vegetable fruits (aubergine, courgette, cucumber, marrow, peppers, pumpkins, squashes, tomatoes) – average	0.9	17	0.3	13	32	6	62	3.9	70	1.5	21	25
Avocados	1.9	4	19.5	92	12	79	9	1.9	4	3.4	190	276
Okra	2.8	35	1.0	29	30	10	30	3.0	36	4.5	31	16
Olives	0.9	3	11.0	96	15	52	12	tr	n	4.0	103	31

Notes: Compared with the average, squash is lower in protein and fat.

Food	Protein grams[1]	% [2]	Total fat grams[1]	% [2]	sfa[3]	mufa[3]	pufa[3]	Carbohydrate grams[1]	% [2]	Fibre grams[1]	Energy per 100g	per portion
7b. Sweet fruits												
Apples and pears – average	0.4	4	0.1	2	n	n	n	10.4	94	2.2	41	62
Melons – average	0.6	8	0.2	6	n	n	n	6.3	86	0.6	28	49
Tropical (mango, pawpaw, banana, pineapple) – average	0.7	5	0.2	3	n	n	n	14.1	92	2.4	57	68
Lychees	0.9	6	0.1	2	n	n	n	14.3	92	1.5	58	28

1 Grams per hundred grams of food.
2 Percentage of total energy.
3 sfa = saturated fatty acid, mufa = monounsaturated fatty acid, pufa = polyunsaturated fatty acid.
4 n = figures not available.

Table 1. Protein, Fat, Carbohydrate, Fibre and Energy

Food	Protein grams[1]	%[2]	Total fat grams[1]	%[2]	Fatty acids as % of total fat sfa[3]	mufa[3]	pufa[3]	Carbohydrate grams[1]	%[2]	Fibre grams[1]	Energy (kilocalories) per 100g	per portion
7b. Sweet fruits, contd.												
Soft fruits (apricots, peaches, plums, greengages, damsons, nectarines, sharon fruit, grapes, cherries) – average	0.8	7	0.1	2	n[4]	n	n	10.8	91	2.1	44	44
Kiwi	1.1	9	0.5	9	n	n	n	10.6	82	1.9	49	29
7c. Citrus fruits (clementines, grapefruits, lemons, oranges, satsumas, tangerines) – average	0.9	10	0.1	3	n	n	n	8.1	87	1.7	35	28
Notes: Lemons are higher than the average in fat. A normal portion of lemon is much lower than the average in calories.												
7d. Dried fruits (apricots, dates, figs, prunes, raisins, sultanas) – average	3.2	6	0.6	2	n	n	n	56.9	92	11.5	232	70
8. Berries												
8a. Blackberries, blackcurrants, cranberries, gooseberries, raspberries, redcurrants, strawberries – average	0.9	14	0.2	5	n	n	n	5.6	81	5.3	26	20
9. Fungi												
9a. All types of mushroom – average	1.8	55	0.5	34	30	2	69	0.4	11	2.3	13	7

1 Grams per hundred grams of food.
2 Percentage of total energy.
3 sfa = saturated fatty acid, mufa = monounsaturated fatty acid, pufa = polyunsaturated fatty acid.
4 n = figures not available.

Table 1. Protein, Fat, Carbohydrate, Fibre and Energy

Food	Protein grams[1]	%[2]	Total fat grams[1]	%[2]	Fatty acids as % of total fat sfa[3]	mufa[3]	pufa[3]	Carbohydrate grams[1]	%[2]	Fibre grams[1]	Energy (kilocalories) per 100g	per portion
10. Oils												
10a. Oils high in SFA (coconut and palm oils) – average	tr[5]	–	99.9	–	67	22	6	0.0	–	–	899	135
10b. Oils high in MUFA (hazelnut, olive and peanut oil) – average	tr	–	99.9	–	14	65	17	0.0	–	–	899	135
10c. Oils high in PUFA (corn, evening primrose, grapeseed, safflower, sesame, soya, sunflower, wheatgerm, mixed vegetable oil) – average	tr	–	99.9	–	13	34	49	0.0	–	–	899	135
11. Miscellaneous Plant Products												
11a. Yeast extract	40.7	91	0.4	2	n[4]	n	n	3.5	7	n	180	7
11b. Soy sauce	3.0	28	tr	n	tr	tr	tr	8.2	72	n	43	6
11c. Vinegar	0.4	–	0.0	0	0	0	0	0.6	–	n	22	3
11d. Seaweeds	1.5	75	0.2	23	n	n	n	tr	–	12.3	8	4

1 Grams per hundred grams of food.
2 Percentage of total energy.
3 sfa = saturated fatty acid, mufa = monounsaturated fatty acid, pufa = polyunsaturated fatty acid.
4 n = figures not available.
5 tr = trace.

199

NUTRITIONAL CONTENTS OF PLANT FOODS

Table 2. Minerals and Trace Elements (per 100g)

Food	Sodium mg	Potassium mg	Calcium mg	Magnesium mg	Phosporus mg	Iron mg	Copper mg	Zinc mg	Sulphur mg	Manganese mg	Selenium µg	Iodine µg
1. Roots and Tubers												
1a. Beetroot, carrots, celeriac, parsnips, swedes, turnips – average	37	307	37	12	44	0.5	0.02	0.2	18	0.2	1	2
1b. Potatoes – average	8	297	6	15	33	0.4	0.07	0.2	25	0.1	1	3
Sweet potatoes	52	480	31	23	65	0.9	0.18	0.4	17	0.5	1	3
Yams	3	510	20	20	36	0.9	0.01	0.4	19	0.1	n	n
1c. Fresh ginger	10	320	18	35	29	0.8	n	0.4	n	n	n	n
1d. Horseradish	8	580	120	36	70	2.0	0.23	1.4	210	0.5	n	n
1e. Radishes	11	240	19	5	20	0.6	0.01	0.2	38	0.1	2	1
2. Bulbs												
2a. Onions, shallots, spring onions, leeks – average	7	208	24	6	37	1.0	0.04	0.3	53	0.1	1	3
2b. Garlic	4	620	19	25	170	1.9	0.06	1.0	n¹	0.5	2	3
3. Stems												
3a. Celery and fennel – average	36	380	33	7	24	0.4	0.02	0.3	15	0.1	3	n

Notes: *Compared with the average, onions are lower in iron; spring onions are higher in calcium.*

1 n = figures not available.

Table 2. Minerals and Trace Elements (per 100g)

Food	Sodium mg	Potassium mg	Calcium mg	Magnesium mg	Phosporus mg	Iron mg	Copper mg	Zinc mg	Sulphur mg	Manganese mg	Selenium µg	Iodine µg
4. Leaves												
4a. Greens – (brussels sprouts, cabbage, curly kale, endive, spinach, spring greens) – average	17	403	105	22	64	1.8	0.02	0.4	48	0.4	1	2
Notes: Spinach is higher than the average in sodium.												
4b. Salads (all lettuces) – average	3	220	28	6	28	0.7	0.01	0.2	16	0.3	1	2
4c. Cress (mustard and cress, watercress) – average	34	170	110	19	43	1.6	0.01	0.5	135	0.6	n[1]	n
4d. Herbs (basil, chives, coriander, dill, mint, oregano, parsley, rosemary, sage, tarragon, thyme) – average	19	415	266	42	50	5.4	n	1.0	n	0.8	n	n
Notes: Compared with the average, chives, oregano and sage are lower in sodium; coriander is lower in zinc; mint is higher in selenium; sage is higher in calcium, magnesium and manganese; thyme is higher in zinc.												
5. Flowers												
5a. Artichoke, green broccoli, purple broccoli, cauliflower – average	7	350	36	20	64	1.1	0.05	0.6	91	0.2	tr[2]	2
Notes: Compared with the average, artichoke is higher in sodium and lower in sulphur; purple broccoli is higher in calcium.												

1 n = figures not available.
2 tr = trace.

Table 2. Minerals and Trace Elements (per 100g)

Food	Sodium mg	Potassium mg	Calcium mg	Magnesium mg	Phosporus mg	Iron mg	Copper mg	Zinc mg	Sulphur mg	Manganese mg	Selenium µg	Iodine µg
6. Seeds												
6a. Pulses												
Fresh pulses (broad beans, runner beans, mange tout, sugar snap and ordinary peas) – average	2	240	35	25	75	1.0	0.06	0.6	33	0.3	n[1]	3
Mung beans sprouts	5	74	20	18	48	1.7	0.08	0.3	n	0.3	n	n
Alfalfa sprouts	6	79	32	27	70	1.0	0.16	0.9	n	0.2	n	n

Notes: Peas are higher than the average in iron.

Food	Sodium mg	Potassium mg	Calcium mg	Magnesium mg	Phosporus mg	Iron mg	Copper mg	Zinc mg	Sulphur mg	Manganese mg	Selenium µg	Iodine µg
Dried pulses (aduki, black gram, black-eye, butter, haricot, mung, pinto, red kidney beans, chick-peas, dal and split peas) – average	7	362	37	43	116	1.9	0.26	1.1	44	0.5	4	n
Green & brown lentils	3	310	22	34	130	3.5	0.33	1.4	n	0.5	40	n
Red lentils	12	220	16	26	100	2.4	0.19	1.0	39	n	2	n
Soya products (incl. soya beans, tempeh, tofu) – average	4	440	87	52	182	2.6	0.40	1.1	n	0.8	n	n
Soya flour	9	1660	210	240	600	6.9	2.92	3.9	n	2.3	9	n
Soya milk	n	n	n	n	n	n	n	n	n	n	n	n
Baked beans	550	300	48	31	95	1.4	0.04	0.5	43	0.3	2	3
Hummus	670	190	41	62	160	1.9	0.30	1.4	n	0.5	n	n

Notes: Compared with the average, tofu is lower in potassium and higher in magnesium.

1 n = figures not available.

Table 2. Minerals and Trace Elements (per 100g)

6b. Grains

Food	Sodium mg	Potassium mg	Calcium mg	Magnesium mg	Phosporus mg	Iron mg	Copper mg	Zinc mg	Sulphur mg	Manganese mg	Selenium µg	Iodine µg
Wholegrains and flours (barley, buckwheat, bulgur, couscous, millet, rye, wheat) – average	5	334	36	98	273	3.6	0.43	2.5	n[1]	1.5	17	9

Notes: White wheat flour may be fortified with calcium and therefore may contain much more calcium than the average.

Food	Sodium mg	Potassium mg	Calcium mg	Magnesium mg	Phosporus mg	Iron mg	Copper mg	Zinc mg	Sulphur mg	Manganese mg	Selenium µg	Iodine µg
Rice products (brown rice, white rice, basmati) – average	5	180	11	62	161	1.1	0.52	1.6	84	1.6	6	14
Rice flour	5	240	24	23	130	1.9	0.20	n	n	n	n	n
Breads (brown, white, wholemeal, rye) – average	535	175	87	49	145	2.5	0.20	1.2	91	1.1	32	n
Pasta (spaghetti, macaroni, tagliatelle, etc.) – average	8	275	26	52	225	2.4	0.36	1.9	178	0.9	16	tr[2]

Notes: Wholemeal spaghetti is higher than the average in potassium, magnesium and manganese.

Food	Sodium mg	Potassium mg	Calcium mg	Magnesium mg	Phosporus mg	Iron mg	Copper mg	Zinc mg	Sulphur mg	Manganese mg	Selenium µg	Iodine µg
Cereals (muesli)	29	510	49	96	310	3.4	0.36	2.1	n	2.6	n	n
Porridge	560	46	7	18	47	0.5	0.03	0.4	20	0.5	tr	n

Notes: These figures apply to muesli and porridge with no added sugar, and porridge made with water.

Food	Sodium mg	Potassium mg	Calcium mg	Magnesium mg	Phosporus mg	Iron mg	Copper mg	Zinc mg	Sulphur mg	Manganese mg	Selenium µg	Iodine µg
Wheat bran	28	1160	110	520	1200	12.9	1.34	16.3	65	9.0	2	n
Cornflour	52	61	15	7	39	1.4	0.13	0.3	–	n	n	n
Corn-on-the-cob	1	150	2	21	53	0.4	0.02	0.2	n	0.1	tr	n
Oatmeal	33	370	55	110	380	4.1	0.23	3.3	160	3.7	3	n
Oatcakes	510	320	48	98	330	3.6	0.20	2.9	142	3.2	3	n
Sago	3	5	10	3	29	1.2	0.03	n	–	n	n	n
Semolina	12	170	18	32	110	1.0	0.15	0.6	92	0.6	n	n
Wheatgerm	5	950	55	270	1050	8.5	0.90	17.0	250	12.3	3	n

1 n = figures not available.
2 tr = trace.

Table 2. Minerals and Trace Elements (per 100g)

Food	Sodium mg	Potassium mg	Calcium mg	Magnesium mg	Phosporus mg	Iron mg	Copper mg	Zinc mg	Sulphur mg	Manganese mg	Selenium µg	Iodine µg
6c. Spices (anise, caraway, celery, coriander, cumin, dill, fennel, mustard seed) – average	69	1384	1030	315	505	32.9	1.06	4.8	n[1]	3.4	n	n

Notes: *Compared with the average, coriander is lower in iron; mustard is lower in sodium, potassium and copper.*

Food	Sodium mg	Potassium mg	Calcium mg	Magnesium mg	Phosporus mg	Iron mg	Copper mg	Zinc mg	Sulphur mg	Manganese mg	Selenium µg	Iodine µg
6d. Nuts and seeds (almonds, brazils, cashews, hazels, pecans and walnuts, pine kernels, pumpkin, sesame and sunflower seeds) – average	8	679	167	265	543	3.5	1.40	4.3	205	2.6	14	12

Notes: *Compared with the average, brazil nuts are higher in selenium; pine kernels are higher in manganese; pumpkin seeds and sesame seeds are higher in iron.*

7. Fruits

Food	Sodium mg	Potassium mg	Calcium mg	Magnesium mg	Phosporus mg	Iron mg	Copper mg	Zinc mg	Sulphur mg	Manganese mg	Selenium µg	Iodine µg
7a. Vegetable fruits (aubergine, courgette, cucumber, marrow, peppers, pumpkin, squash, tomatoes) – average	3	221	20	16	28	0.5	0.03	0.2	17	0.1	1	2

Notes: *Marrow is lower than the average in sulphur.*

Food	Sodium mg	Potassium mg	Calcium mg	Magnesium mg	Phosporus mg	Iron mg	Copper mg	Zinc mg	Sulphur mg	Manganese mg	Selenium µg	Iodine µg
Avocados	6	450	11	25	39	0.4	0.19	0.4	19	0.2	tr[2]	2
Okra	8	330	160	71	59	1.1	0.13	0.6	30	n	1	n
Olives	2250	91	61	22	17	1.0	0.23	n	36	n	n	n
7b. Sweet fruits												
Apples and pears – average	3	131	8	6	12	0.2	0.04	0.1	5	0.1	tr	1
Melons – average	13	145	11	10	11	0.3	n	0.1	9	tr	tr	tr
Tropical (mango, pawpaw, banana, pineapple) – average	3	235	15	19	17	0.4	0.10	0.2	10	0.3	n	n

1 n = figures not available.
2 tr = trace.

Table 2. Minerals and Trace Elements (per 100g)

Food	Sodium mg	Potassium mg	Calcium mg	Magnesium mg	Phosporus mg	Iron mg	Copper mg	Zinc mg	Sulphur mg	Manganese mg	Selenium µg	Iodine µg
7b. Sweet fruits, contd.												
Kiwi	4	290	25	15	32	0.4	0.13	0.1	16	0.1	n[1]	n
Lychees	1	160	6	9	30	0.5	0.15	0.3	19	0.1	n	n
Soft fruits (apricots, peaches, plums, greengages, damsons, nectarines, sharon fruit, grapes, cherries) – average	2	227	13	9	20	0.3	0.08	0.1	6	0.1	1	2
7c. Citrus fruits (clementines, grapefruits, lemons, oranges, satsumas, tangerines) – average	4	152	34	10	18	0.2	0.02	0.1	9	tr[2]	1	n
7d. Dried fruits (apricots, dates, figs, prunes, raisins, sultanas) – average	37	1082	57	47	86	3.1	0.32	0.6	44	0.4	5	n

Notes: *Compared with the average, apricots are higher in sodium and sulphur; figs are higher in calcium.*

8. Berries

Food	Sodium mg	Potassium mg	Calcium mg	Magnesium mg	Phosporus mg	Iron mg	Copper mg	Zinc mg	Sulphur mg	Manganese mg	Selenium µg	Iodine µg
8a. Blackberries, blackcurrants, cranberries, gooseberries, raspberries, redcurrants, strawberries – average	3	201	25	14	27	0.8	0.09	0.2	18	0.4	tr	n

Notes: *Blackcurrants are higher than the average in calcium.*

9. Fungi

Food	Sodium mg	Potassium mg	Calcium mg	Magnesium mg	Phosporus mg	Iron mg	Copper mg	Zinc mg	Sulphur mg	Manganese mg	Selenium µg	Iodine µg
9a. All types of mushroom – average	5	320	6	9	80	0.6	0.72	0.4	34	0.1	9	3

1 n = figures not available.
2 tr = trace.

Table 2. Minerals and Trace Elements (per 100g)

Food	Sodium mg	Potassium mg	Calcium mg	Magnesium mg	Phosporus mg	Iron mg	Copper mg	Zinc mg	Sulphur mg	Manganese mg	Selenium µg	Iodine µg
10. Oils												
10a. Oils high in SFA (coconut and palm oil) – average	tr[1]	tr	tr	tr	tr	tr	tr	tr	tr	tr	tr	tr
10b. Oils high in MUFA (hazelnut, olive and peanut oil) – average	tr	tr	tr	tr	tr	tr	tr	tr	tr	tr	tr	tr
10c. Oils high in PUFA (corn, evening primrose, grapeseed, safflower, sesame, soya, sunflower, wheatgerm, mixed vegetable oil) – average	tr	tr	tr	tr	tr	tr	tr	tr	tr	tr	tr	tr
11. Miscellaneous Plant Products												
11a. Yeast extract	4300	2100	70	160	950	2.9	0.20	2.7	n[2]	0.2	n	49
11b. Soy sauce	7120	180	17	37	47	2.4	0.01	0.2	n	0.2	n	n
11c. Vinegar	5	34	3	4	10	0.1	0.01	0.1	n	0.0	1	n
11d. Seaweeds	67	63	72	n	160	8.9	0.15	1.9	n	0.4	n	n

1 tr = trace.
2 n = figures not available.

NUTRITIONAL CONTENTS OF PLANT FOODS

Table 3. Vitamins (per 100g)

Food	Vitamin A[1] µg	Vitamin E mg	Thiamin mg	Riboflavin mg	Niacin mg	Niacin from Tryptophan[2] mg	Vitamin B6 mg	Folate µg	Pantothenate mg	Biotin µg	Vitamin C mg
1. Roots and Tubers											
1a. Beetroot, carrots, celeriac, parsnips, swedes, turnips – average	4	0.70	0.11	0.01	0.5	0.2	0.10	37	0.24	0.3	13
1b. Potatoes – average	tr[3]	0.04	0.15	0.05	0.4	0.4	0.32	23	0.34	0.3	8
Sweet potatoes	857	5.96	0.09	tr	0.5	0.3	0.07	9	0.59	n[4]	23
Yams	tr	n	0.17	0.01	0.2	0.4	0.15	7	0.38	n	5
1c. Fresh ginger	8	n	0.01	0.03	0.8	n	0.16	n	0.20	n	4
1d. Horseradish	0	tr	0.05	0.03	0.5	0.7	0.15	n	n	n	120
1e. Radishes	tr	0.00	0.03	tr	0.4	0.1	0.07	38	0.18	n	17

Notes: Compared with the average, beetroot is higher in folic acid; carrots and swedes are much higher in vitamin A (1 portion of carrots contains more than 800 µg of vitamin A.)

Food	Vitamin A[1] µg	Vitamin E mg	Thiamin mg	Riboflavin mg	Niacin mg	Niacin from Tryptophan[2] mg	Vitamin B6 mg	Folate µg	Pantothenate mg	Biotin µg	Vitamin C mg
2. Bulbs											
2a. Onions, shallots, spring onions, leeks – average	2	0.50	0.24	0.06	0.6	0.3	0.27	17	0.11	1.0	18
2b. Garlic	tr	0.01	0.13	0.03	0.3	1.9	0.38	5	n	n	17

Notes: Compared with the average, leek is higher in vitamin A and folate; onion is lower in vitamin C; shallot is lower in thiamin.

Food	Vitamin A[1] µg	Vitamin E mg	Thiamin mg	Riboflavin mg	Niacin mg	Niacin from Tryptophan[2] mg	Vitamin B6 mg	Folate µg	Pantothenate mg	Biotin µg	Vitamin C mg
3. Stems											
3a. Celery and fennel – average	16	0.20	0.06	0.01	0.5	0.1	0.05	29	0.40	0.1	7

1 Retinol equivalent – this figure is calculated by dividing the beta-carotene content by 6.
2 The amino acid tryptophan may be converted in the body to niacin. The conversion used here is tryptophan/60 = niacin.
3 tr = trace.
4 n = no figures available.

Table 3. Vitamins (per 100g)

Food	Vitamin A[1] µg	Vitamin E mg	Thiamin mg	Riboflavin mg	Niacin mg	Niacin from Tryptophan[2] mg	Vitamin B6 mg	Folate µg	Pantothenate mg	Biotin µg	Vitamin C mg
4. Leaves											
4a. Greens – brussels sprouts, cabbage, curly kale, endive, spinach, spring greens – average	58	1.47	0.10	0.10	0.8	0.5	0.24	119	0.55	0.4	114
Notes: Compared with the average, cabbage is lower in vitamin E and riboflavin; curly kale is higher in vitamin A and lower in vitamin B6 and C; spinach is higher in vitamin A and lower in vitamin C; spring greens are higher in vitamin A.											
4b. Salads (all lettuces) – average	59	0.57	0.12	0.02	0.4	0.1	0.04	55	0.18	0.7	5
4c. Cress (mustard and cress, watercress) – average	317	1.08	0.10	0.05	0.7	0.4	0.19	60	0.10	0.4	48
4d. Herbs (basil, chives, coriander, dill, mint, oregano, parsley, rosemary, sage, tarragon, thyme) – average	279	1.70	0.12	0.26	1.1	0.5	0.16	n[3]	n	n	46
Notes: Compared with the average, dill is higher in vitamin A; mint is higher in vitamin E; parsley is higher in vitamin C; tarragon is lower in vitamins A and C.											
5. Flowers											
5a. Artichoke, green broccoli, purple broccoli, cauliflower – average	88	1.25	0.12	0.07	1.0	0.7	0.16	199	0.37	0.8	80
Notes: Compared with the average, artichoke is higher in biotin and lower in vitamins A, E and C; purple broccoli is higher in pantothenate and lower in niacin; cauliflower is lower in vitamins A and E.											

1 Retinol equivalent – this figure is calculated by dividing the beta-carotene content by 6.
2 The amino acid tryptophan may be converted in the body to niacin. The conversion used here is tryptophan/60 = niacin.
3 n = no figures available.

Table 3. Vitamins (per 100g)

Food	Vitamin A[1] µg	Vitamin E mg	Thiamin mg	Riboflavin mg	Niacin mg	Niacin from Tryptophan[2] mg	Vitamin B6 mg	Folate µg	Pantothenate mg	Biotin µg	Vitamin C mg
6. Seeds											
6a. Pulses											
Fresh pulses (broad beans, runner beans, mange tout, sugar snap and ordinary peas) – average	51	0.30	0.11	0.08	1.6	0.7	0.11	67	0.10	1.2	29
Mung bean sprouts	7	n[3]	0.11	0.04	0.5	0.5	0.10	61	0.38	n	7
Alfalfa sprouts	16	n	0.04	0.06	0.5	0.6	0.03	36	0.56	n	2
Notes: Compared with the average, broad beans are higher in pantothenate and folate; mange tout are lower in folate and higher in pantothenate and biotin; sugar-snap beans are lower in folate.											
Dried pulses (aduki, black gram, black-eye, butter, haricot, mung, pinto and red kidney beans; chick-peas, dal and split peas) – average	3	0.24	0.13	0.06	0.6	1.3	0.12	50	0.33	n	n
Green & brown lentils	n	n	0.14	0.08	0.6	1.2	0.28	30	n	n	tr
Red lentils	3	n	0.11	0.04	0.4	1.0	0.11	5	0.31	n	tr
Soya products (incl. soya beans, tempeh and tofu) – average	4	n	0.13	0.06	0.3	3.6	0.17	52	0.16	39.0	tr
Soya flour	n	1.50	0.75	0.28	2.0	8.6	0.46	345	1.60	n	0
Soya milk	n	n	n	n	n	n	n	n	n	n	n
Baked beans	12	0.36	0.08	0.06	0.5	0.8	0.12	33	0.18	2.5	tr
Hummus	n	n	0.16	0.05	1.1	1.0	n	n	n	n	1
Notes: Compared with the average, tempeh is higher in vitamin A, riboflavin, niacin, vitamin B6 and pantothenate.											

1 Retinol equivalent – this figure is calculated by dividing the beta-carotene content by 6.
2 The amino acid tryptophan may be converted in the body to niacin. The conversion used here is tryptophan/60 = niacin.
3 n = no figures available.
4 tr = trace.

Table 3. Vitamins (per 100g)

Food	Vitamin A¹ µg	Vitamin E mg	Thiamin mg	Riboflavin mg	Niacin mg	Niacin from Tryptophan² mg	Vitamin B6 mg	Folate µg	Pantothenate mg	Biotin µg	Vitamin C mg
6b. Grains											
Grains and flours (barley, buckwheat, bulgur, couscous, millet, rye, wheat) – average	n³	1.10	0.42	0.12	3.2	1.9	0.39	52	0.80	6.0	0
Rice products (brown rice, white rice, basmati) – average	0	0.50	0.34	0.05	3.4	1.5	0.30	35	0.60	3.0	0
Rice flour	0	n	0.10	0.05	2.1	1.4	0.20	n	n	n	0
Breads (brown, white, wholemeal, rye) – average	0	n	0.28	0.07	2.8	1.8	0.09	36	0.43	3.4	0
Pasta (spaghetti, macaroni, tagliatelle, etc.) – average	0	tr⁴	0.30	0.06	2.8	2.5	0.13	34	0.30	1.0	0

Notes: Wholemeal spagetti is higher than the average in thiamine, riboflavin, B6 and pantothenate

Food	Vitamin A¹ µg	Vitamin E mg	Thiamin mg	Riboflavin mg	Niacin mg	Niacin from Tryptophan² mg	Vitamin B6 mg	Folate µg	Pantothenate mg	Biotin µg	Vitamin C mg
Cereals (muesli)	tr	3.20	0.30	0.30	5.3	2.2	n	n	n	n	tr
Porridge	0	0.21	0.06	0.01	0.1	0.3	0.01	4	0.10	2.0	0

Notes: These figures apply to muesli and porridge with no added sugar, and porridge made with water.

Food	Vitamin A¹ µg	Vitamin E mg	Thiamin mg	Riboflavin mg	Niacin mg	Niacin from Tryptophan² mg	Vitamin B6 mg	Folate µg	Pantothenate mg	Biotin µg	Vitamin C mg
Wheat bran	0	2.60	0.89	0.36	29.6	3.0	1.38	260	2.40	45.0	0
Cornflour	0	tr	tr	tr	tr	0.1	tr	tr	tr	tr	0
Corn-on-the-cob	9	0.40	0.09	0.03	1.1	0.2	0.09	24	0.42	n	5
Oatmeal	0	1.70	0.50	0.10	1.0	2.8	0.12	60	1.00	20.0	0
Oatcakes	0	1.48	0.33	0.07	0.8	2.4	0.08	26	0.70	17.0	0
Sago	0	tr	tr	tr	tr	tr	tr	tr	tr	tr	0
Semolina	0	tr	0.10	0.03	0.7	2.2	0.15	22	0.30	1.0	0
Wheatgerm	0	22.00	2.01	0.72	4.5	5.3	3.30	331	1.90	25.0	0

1 Retinol equivalent – this figure is calculated by dividing the beta-carotene content by 6.
2 The amino acid tryptophan may be converted in the body to niacin. The conversion used here is tryptophan/60 = niacin.
3 n = no figures available.
4 tr = trace.

Table 3. Vitamins (per 100g)

Food	Vitamin A[1] µg	Vitamin E mg	Thiamin mg	Riboflavin mg	Niacin mg	Niacin from Tryptophan[2] mg	Vitamin B6 mg	Folate µg	Pantothenate mg	Biotin µg	Vitamin C mg
6c. Spices (anise, caraway, celery, coriander, cumin, dill, fennel, mustard) – average	8	n[3]	0.43	0.34	3.0	n	n	0	n	n	0

Notes: Compared with the average, caraway and cumin are higher in vitamin A; dill is higher in niacin; mustard is higher in niacin and tryptophan.

Food	Vitamin A[1] µg	Vitamin E mg	Thiamin mg	Riboflavin mg	Niacin mg	Niacin from Tryptophan[2] mg	Vitamin B6 mg	Folate µg	Pantothenate mg	Biotin µg	Vitamin C mg
6d. Nuts and seeds (almonds, brazils, cashews, hazels, pecans and walnuts, pine kernels, pumpkins, sesame and sunflower seeds) – average	1	15.20	0.57	0.29	3.5	4.3	0.43	63	1.36	45.0	0

Notes: Compared with the average, brazil nuts are lower in riboflavin and niacin; pumpkin seeds are higher in vitamin A; sunflower seeds are higher in thiamin.

7. Fruits

Food	Vitamin A[1] µg	Vitamin E mg	Thiamin mg	Riboflavin mg	Niacin mg	Niacin from Tryptophan[2] mg	Vitamin B6 mg	Folate µg	Pantothenate mg	Biotin µg	Vitamin C mg
7a. Vegetable fruits (aubergine, courgette, cucumber, marrow, peppers, pumpkin, squash, tomatoes) – average	50	1.14	0.08	0.02	0.5	0.2	0.14	22	0.22	0.7	13
Avocados	3	3.20	0.10	0.18	1.1	0.3	0.36	11	1.10	3.6	6
Okra	86	n	0.20	0.06	1.0	0.4	0.21	88	0.25	n	21
Olives	30	1.99	tr[4]	tr	tr	0.1	0.02	tr	0.02	tr	0

Notes: Compared with the average, aubergine and cucumber are lower in vitamin E; green and red peppers are higher in vitamin C; red pepper and butternut squash are higher in vitamin A.

1 Retinol equivalent – this figure is calculated by dividing the beta-carotene content by 6.
2 The amino acid tryptophan may be converted in the body to niacin. The conversion used here is tryptophan/60 = niacin.
3 n = no figures available.
4 tr = trace.

Table 3. Vitamins (per 100g)

Food	Vitamin A[1] µg	Vitamin E mg	Thiamin mg	Riboflavin mg	Niacin mg	Niacin from Tryptophan[2] mg	Vitamin B6 mg	Folate µg	Pantothenate mg	Biotin µg	Vitamin C mg
7b. Sweet fruits											
Apples and pears – average	3	0.50	0.03	0.03	0.2	0.1	0.04	3	0.07	0.7	10
Melons – average	61	0.10	0.04	0.01	0.3	tr[3]	0.12	3	0.19	1.0	13
Tropical (mango, pawpaw, banana, pineapple) – average	110	0.50	0.05	0.05	0.5	0.1	0.14	7	0.23	1.5	30
Kiwi	6	n[4]	0.01	0.03	0.3	0.3	0.15	n	n	n	57
Lychees	0	n	0.04	0.06	0.5	0.1	n	n	n	n	45

Notes: *Compared with the average, mango is higher in vitamins A and E; banana is lower in vitamin A; pineapple is lower in vitamins A and E.*

Food	Vitamin A[1] µg	Vitamin E mg	Thiamin mg	Riboflavin mg	Niacin mg	Niacin from Tryptophan[2] mg	Vitamin B6 mg	Folate µg	Pantothenate mg	Biotin µg	Vitamin C mg
Soft fruits (apricots, peaches, plums, greengages, damsons, nectarines, sharon fruit, grapes, cherries) – average	41	0.50	0.04	0.04	0.5	0.1	0.05	4	0.21	0.2	13

Notes: *Grapes are lower than the average in pantothenate.*

Food	Vitamin A[1] µg	Vitamin E mg	Thiamin mg	Riboflavin mg	Niacin mg	Niacin from Tryptophan[2] mg	Vitamin B6 mg	Folate µg	Pantothenate mg	Biotin µg	Vitamin C mg
7c. Citrus fruits (clementines, grapefruits, lemons, oranges, satsumas, tangerines) – average	10	0.20	0.08	0.03	0.3	0.1	0.07	26	0.24	1.0	42

Notes: *Lemon is lower than the average in vitamin A.*

Food	Vitamin A[1] µg	Vitamin E mg	Thiamin mg	Riboflavin mg	Niacin mg	Niacin from Tryptophan[2] mg	Vitamin B6 mg	Folate µg	Pantothenate mg	Biotin µg	Vitamin C mg
7d. Dried fruits (apricots, dates, figs, prunes, raisins, sultanas) – average	5	n	0.09	0.12	1.1	0.4	0.23	10	0.52	3.4	tr

Notes: *Compared with the average, apricots and prunes are higher in vitamin A; dates are higher in tryptophan; raisins and sultanas are lower in pantothenate; sultanas are higher in folate.*

1 Retinol equivalent – this figure is calculated by dividing the beta-carotene content by 6.
2 The amino acid tryptophan may be converted in the body to niacin. The conversion used here is tryptophan/60 = niacin.
3 tr = trace.
4 n = no figures available.

Table 3. Vitamins (per 100g)

Food	Vitamin A[1] µg	Vitamin E mg	Thiamin mg	Riboflavin mg	Niacin mg	Niacin from Tryptophan[2] mg	Vitamin B6 mg	Folate µg	Pantothenate mg	Biotin µg	Vitamin C mg
8. Berries											
8a. Blackberries, blackcurrants, cranberries, gooseberries, raspberries, redcurrants, strawberries – average	10	0.40	0.03	0.04	0.3	0.1	0.06	24	0.29	2.0	34
9. Fungi											
9a. All types of mushroom – average	0	0.12	0.09	0.31	3.2	0.3	0.18	44	2.00	12.0	1
10. Oils											
10a. Oils high in SFA (coconut and palm oil) – average	tr[3]	n[4]	tr	tr	tr	tr	tr	tr	tr	tr	0
10b. Oils high in MUFA (hazelnut, olive and peanut oil) – average	tr	n	tr	tr	tr	tr	tr	tr	tr	tr	0
10c. Oils high in PUFA (corn, evening primrose, grapeseed, safflower, sesame, soya, sunflower, wheatgerm, mixed vegetable oil) – average	tr	n	tr	tr	tr	tr	tr	tr	tr	tr	0

Notes: Compared with the average, blackberries are higher in vitamin E and lower in pantothenate; blackcurrants are higher in vitamin C; cranberries are lower in folate; gooseberries are lower in biotin; raspberries and strawberries are lower in vitamin A; redcurrants are lower in pantothenate.

Notes: All vegetable oils contain vitamin E, but there are large variations in the amounts. An average is therefore not given.

1 Retinol equivalent – this figure is calculated by dividing the beta-carotene content by 6.
2 The amino acid tryptophan may be converted in the body to niacin. The conversion used here is tryptophan/60 = niacin.
3 tr = trace.
4 n = no figures available.

Table 3. Vitamins (per 100g)

Food	Vitamin A[1] µg	Vitamin E mg	Thiamin mg	Riboflavin mg	Niacin mg	Niacin from Tryptophan[2] mg	Vitamin B6 mg	Folate µg	Pantothenate mg	Biotin µg	Vitamin C mg
11. Miscellaneous Plant Products											
11a. Yeast extract	0	n[3]	4.10	11.90	64.0	9.0	1.60	1150	n	n	0
11b. Soy sauce	0	n	0.05	0.13	3.4	1.4	n	11	n	n	0
11c. Vinegar	0	0	0.00	0.00	0.0	0.0	0.00	0	0	0	0
11d. Seaweeds	n	n	0.01	0.47	0.6	n	n	n	0.18	n	n

1 Retinol equivalent – this figure is calculated by dividing the beta-carotene content by 6.
2 The amino acid tryptophan may be converted in the body to niacin. The conversion used here is tryptophan/60 = niacin.
3 n = no figures available.

VITAMINS

Vitamins are divided into two groups or classes – those that dissolve in water and those that dissolve in oil and fat.

The water-soluble vitamins are:

The B group

B1 or thiamin	B12 or cobalamin
B2 or riboflavin	Folate (folic acid)
B3 or niacin	Pantothenic acid
B6 or pyridoxine	Biotin

Vitamin C

The fat-soluble vitamins are:

Vitamin A
Beta-carotene (plants)
Retinol (animals)

Vitamin D
D2 or ergocalciferol (plants)
D3 or cholecalciferol (animals)

Vitamin E
Tocopherols

Vitamin K
Coagulation vitamin

Vitamins are essential to health, although they are needed only in very small amounts. Most of them are obtained from the food we eat, but some are made within the body. Vitamin D is produced by skin exposed to daylight.

Vitamin B3 is made in body cells out of the amino-acid tryptophan. Vitamin K, biotin, pantothenic acid and vitamin B12 can be synthesized by bacteria that live in the intestines.

This appendix describes each vitamin in turn and, as fresh fruits, nuts, vegetables, pulses and grains are particularly rich in vitamins, the twenty top plant sources of each vitamin are also listed, ranked according to vitamin content per average *portion*. If you should want to increase your intake of any particular vitamin, it is important to know how much of it you can expect to get from an amount of food you are actually likely to be able to eat. The common practice of quoting nutrient contents only in terms of content per 100 grams is often misleading in this respect.

Note When reading the deficiency sections below, it may help to remember that vitamin deficiency has three basic causes:

1. Not enough is being eaten.
2. Not enough is being absorbed.
3. Bodily demand is outstripping dietary supply.

Vitamin deficiencies are rare in Western society, except in people suffering from serious chronic disease.

Water soluble vitamins – the B-group

Vitamin B1 – Thiamin

Background Thiamin is found in all unprocessed foods. However, the refining of cereals (to produce white flour, for example) removes thiamin, and therefore many cereal products are fortified with vitamin B1. Cooking, particularly prolonged boiling, causes some loss of thiamin from food.

Importance Thiamin plays an essential role in the process by which the body makes use of the energy contained in carbohydrates, fats and alcohol. The more carbohydrate, fat and alcohol we consume, the more thiamin we need.

Deficiency Vitamin B1 deficiency is associated with alcoholism, severe malnutrition, serious chronic disease and intestinal conditions that interfere with the absorption of nutrients. It results in the condition known as 'beri-beri', which produces muscle weakness, nerve problems and, eventually, heart failure. In alcoholism, thiamin deficiency may produce a syndrome of disturbed balance, confusion and memory loss.

Toxicity Thiamin has no known adverse effects (except when given in high doses by injection).

20 good sources of Thiamin (B1) found in common plant foods

	Portion size (g)	Food	mg per 100g	mg per portion
1	90	Peas	.74	.67
2	150	Brown rice	.30	.45
3	10	Yeast extract	4.10	.41
4	180	Potatoes	.21	.38
5	50	Muesli	.50	.25
6	15	Sunflower seeds	1.60	.24
7	90	Pinto beans	.23	.21
8	90	Cabbage	.22	.20
9	20	Tahini paste	.94	.19
10	60	Leeks	.29	.17
11	15	Peanuts	1.14	.17
12	30	Wheatgerm bread	.52	.16
13	20	Soya flour	.75	.15
14	30	Malt bread	.45	.14
15	20	Millet flour	.68	.14
16	60	Parsnips	.23	.14
17	15	Sesame seeds	.93	.14
18	30	Brown rolls	.43	.13
19	15	Pecan nuts	.71	.11
20	15	Pistachio nuts	.70	.11

Vitamin B2 – Riboflavin

Background Riboflavin is found in most natural foods, but cooking destroys up to forty percent of it.

Importance Like thiamin, riboflavin is needed in the body to help release the energy from food.

Deficiency Riboflavin deficiency is not common, but may occur in alcoholism, diabetes, anorexia, severe malnutrition and diseases that cause malabsorption. The symptoms are cracks at the corners of the mouth, sore tongue and a rash around the nose.

Toxicity Riboflavin has no known toxic effects.

20 good sources of Riboflavin (B2) found in common plant foods

	Portion size (g)	Type	mg per 100g	mg per portion
1	10	Yeast extract	11.90	1.19
2	90	Tempeh	.48	.43
3	50	Muesli	.70	.35
4	145	Avocado	.18	.26
5	90	Fenugreek leaves	.28	.25
6	50	Seaweed (Irish moss)	.47	.24
7	50	Oyster mushrooms	.43	.22
8	125	Sweetcorn	.17	.21
9	50	Mushrooms	.31	.16
10	90	Mange tout peas	.15	.14
11	90	Sugar snap peas	.14	.13
12	90	Mustard leaves	.13	.12
13	90	Broccoli, purple	.12	.11
14	15	Almonds	.75	.11
15	90	Brussels sprouts	.11	.10
16	90	Spring greens	.11	.10
17	90	Endive	.10	.09
18	20	Carob flour	.46	.09
19	5	Coriander leaves (fresh)	1.50	.08
20	90	Curly kale	.09	.08

Vitamin B3 – Niacin (nicotinic acid and niacinamide)

Background   Niacin is found in a wide variety of foods. The essential amino acid tryptophan (which is one of the components of the protein we eat) can also be converted by the body into niacin. So, as long as our diet contains sufficient protein, we will cover our niacin requirements independent of the amount of B3 in our food.

Importance   Vitamin B3 is needed to release energy from food within the body. How much we need of it is related to how much energy we use up each day.

Deficiency   We obtain vitamin B3 from two reliable sources (as niacin in food and from the conversion of tryptophan in protein) and so niacin deficiency is rare, except in cases of severe malnourishment. When it does occur, it causes pellagra, a syndrome consisting of skin rash, weakness, diarrhoea and mental disturbance.

Toxicity High doses of niacin cause flushing of the skin and cause the stomach to secrete excess acid (which increases the risk of stomach ulcers). Very high doses (3 to 6 grams per day) may even cause liver damage.

20 good sources of Niacin (B3) found in common plant foods

	Portion size (g)	Type	B3 (mg) per 100g	Tryptophan per 100g	Total B3 (mg) per portion
1	10	Yeast extract	64.0	9.0	7.3
2	90	Tempeh	3.2	4.7	7.1
3	50	Muesli	6.5	2.3	4.4
4	90	Broad beans	3.2	.9	3.7
5	180	Baked potato	1.1	.9	3.6
6	20	Peanut butter	12.5	4.9	3.5
7	90	Peas	2.5	1.1	3.2
8	15	Peanuts	13.8	5.5	2.9
9	150	Brown rice	1.3	.6	2.9
10	90	Soya beans	.5	2.2	2.4
11	7	Wheat bran	29.6	3.0	2.3
12	90	Aduki beans	.9	1.5	2.2
13	20	Soya flour	2.0	8.6	2.1
14	125	Sweetcorn	1.2	.3	1.9
15	50	Mushrooms	3.2	.3	1.8
16	120	Red pepper	1.3	.2	1.8
17	90	Spring greens	1.5	.5	1.8
18	30	Dried peaches	5.3	.7	1.8
19	30	Wholemeal bread	4.1	1.8	1.8
20	20	Tahini paste	5.1	4.1	1.8

Vitamin B6 – Pyridoxine

Background Pyridoxine is found in many different foods. Freezing and thawing can cause significant B6 loss.

Importance Vitamin B6 plays an important role in protein metabolism and is involved in the conversion of the amino acid tryptophan into niacin (vitamin B3 – see above). The more protein we eat, the more pyridoxine we need. B6 is also necessary for making haemoglobin and for the normal functioning of the nervous system.

Deficiency Vitamin B6 deficiency is rare, but is associated with alcoholism, Parkinson's disease, chronic liver and kidney disease, coeliac disease and some inherited disorders. Some of the drugs used to treat tuberculosis and rheumatoid arthritis interfere with vitamin B6, as does the oral contraceptive pill. There have also been suggestions that vitamin B6 deficiency may be related to epilepsy, asthma and pre-menstrual syndrome.

The symptoms of vitamin B6 deficiency include a skin rash around the eyes, nose and mouth, cracked lips and mouth corners, a sore tongue, migraine, depression, irritability and tiredness. It may also cause disturbance of sensation in the hands and feet.

Toxicity Paradoxically, taking vitamin B6 supplements in excess of 100–200mg per day over long periods may cause serious (though reversible) loss of sensation in the hands and feet.

20 good sources of Pyridoxine (B6) found in common plant foods

	Portion size (g)	Type	mg per 100g	mg per portion
1	90	Tempeh	1.86	1.67
2	50	Muesli	1.60	0.80
3	180	Potatoes	0.44	0.79
4	145	Avocado	0.36	0.52
5	120	Red pepper	0.36	0.43
6	120	Yellow pepper	0.33	0.40
7	120	Green pepper	0.30	0.36
8	120	Bananas	0.29	0.35
9	90	Brussels sprouts	0.37	0.33
10	60	Leeks	0.48	0.29
11	90	Lentils, boiled	0.28	0.25
12	90	Curly kale	0.26	0.23
13	75	Elderberries	0.24	0.18
14	5	Wheat germ	3.30	0.17
15	10	Yeast extract	1.60	0.16
16	20	Tahini paste	0.76	0.15
17	50	Cauliflower	0.28	0.14
18	50	Broccoli, purple	0.25	0.13
19	20	Peanut butter	0.58	0.12
20	7	Wheat bran	1.38	0.10

Vitamin B12 – Cobalamin

Background Vitamin B12 is only required in tiny amounts and is unique amongst vitamins in being produced entirely by micro-organisms living in the soil and in the intestines. Fresh, unprocessed, organically grown vegetables lightly washed in pure water do contain small amounts of harmless soil bacteria and thus some vitamin B12. Modern, sterile, agrochemically produced vegetables contain no vitamin B12.

Importance   Vitamin B12 is necessary, together with folic acid (see below), for the normal growth and development of all rapidly dividing cells; for example, bone marrow (which produces red and white blood cells).

Deficiency   Vitamin B12 deficiency is rare but is seen sometimes in people suffering from malabsorption syndromes, intestinal parasites and alcoholism. It produces a sore tongue, diarrhoea and weakness. B12 deficiency also causes anaemia (pernicious anaemia) and can, over a long period of time, result in damage to the nervous system, particularly the spinal cord. Smokers, and people taking antibiotics, have an increased need for vitamin B12.

Toxicity   There are no known toxic effects of vitamin B12.

Some good sources of Vitamin B12 found in common plant-based foods

Portion size (g)	Type	µg per 100g	µg per portion
	Yeast extracts (f)		
4	Marmite	13.30	0.53
4	Natex	8.80	0.35
	Vegetable stock		
10	Vecon	13.00	1.30
	Vegetable margarines (f)		
7	Granose	5.00	0.35
	Soya milks (f)		
100	Plamil	1.60	1.60
100	Unisoy Gold	0.60	0.60
	Breakfast cereals (f)		
50	Various	2.00	1.00

f = fortified

Folate

Background   Folate is widely available in plant foods and is also found in some animal foods. Cooking, particularly boiling, destroys between twenty and fifty percent of the folate content of food.

Importance   The body uses folate in the manufacture of amino acids and also in the production of DNA. It works with vitamin B12 to support the growth and development of rapidly dividing cells, and can protect against the anaemia caused by vitamin B12 deficiency. Folate seems to be particularly important for the normal development of the nervous system of the baby during pregnancy.

Deficiency   Folate deficiency is not common in the West, but when it does occur it causes anaemia, weakness and depression.

Folate deficiency has three main causes:

1 Malnourishment amongst the elderly, the poor and alcoholics (in the USA, alcoholism is the most common cause of folate deficiency).

2 Poor absorption from the gut, which may be caused by gastro-intestinal disease and some drugs (eg. for epilepsy and inflammatory bowel disease);

3 Increased need, for example during pregnancy and breast feeding (and also in certain blood disorders, such as leukaemia).

In a generally healthy population, the groups most at risk of folate deficiency are the elderly, premature babies and pregnant women (particularly those in the poorest sections of society, who are likely to suffer from poor general nutrition). There also seems to be an association between folate deficiency and the risk of having a baby with a neural tube defect such as spina bifida; this has led to the recommendation of folate supplements to all pregnant mothers. Note that people eating a high proportion of unprocessed and raw vegetables in their diet have a higher than average folate intake.

Toxicity   Folate toxicity is rare, but high doses may interfere with the absorption of zinc from the diet.

20 good sources of Folate found in common plant foods

	Portion size (g)	Type	µg per 100g	µg per portion
1	90	Black-eyed beans	210	189
2	90	Swiss chard	165	149
3	90	Savoy cabbage	150	135
4	90	Spinach	150	135
5	90	Broad beans	145	131
6	90	Pinto beans	145	131
7	90	Endive	140	126
8	90	Brussels sprouts	135	122

	Portion size (g)	Type	µg per 100g	µg per portion
9	90	Curly kale	120	108
10	120	Okra	88	106
11	50	Purple broccoli	195	98
12	60	Beetroot	150	90
13	50	Asparagus	175	88
14	90	Spring greens	92	83
15	90	Green beans	80	72
16	50	Muesli	140	70
17	20	Soya flour	345	69
18	90	Tempeh	76	68
19	90	Cabbage	75	68
20	180	Potatoes	35	63

Pantothenic acid

Background Pantothenic acid is found in a wide variety of foods, and is also produced by bacteria in our intestines. Food processing reduces pantothenic acid content, and pantothenic acid in meat is destroyed by roasting.

Importance Like the other B-group vitamins, pantothenic acid is needed by the body to make use of the energy contained in fats, carbohydrates, protein and alcohol. It is also involved in the production of antibodies, in converting cholesterol into natural steroid hormones, in detoxifying drugs and in maintaining the health of the nervous system. It could be called an anti-stress vitamin.

Deficiency Deficiency of pantothenic acid is rare, but may cause a sensation of burning in the feet and a disturbance of blood pressure control in cases of severe malnourishment. Pantothenic acid deficiency may also be related to allergy.

Toxicity Pantothenic acid appears to have no toxic effects.

20 good sources of Pantothenic acid found in common plant foods

	Portion size (g)	Type	mg per 100g	mg per portion
1	90	Broad beans	4.94	4.45
2	145	Avocado	1.10	1.60

table continues

	Portion size (g)	Type	mg per 100g	mg per portion
3	50	Mushrooms	2.00	1.00
4	90	Tempeh	1.06	.95
5	90	Brussels sprouts	1.00	.90
6	90	Purple broccoli	1.00	.90
7	90	Endive	.90	.81
8	125	Sweetcorn	.63	.79
9	130	Sweet potato	.59	.77
10	180	Potatoes	.37	.67
11	90	Mange tout peas	.72	.65
12	120	Acorn squash	.50	.60
13	20	Tahini paste	2.17	.43
14	15	Peanuts	2.66	.40
15	90	Butter beans, boiled	.42	.38
16	90	Dal, cooked	.41	.37
17	20	Peanut butter	1.70	.34
18	15	Sesame seeds	2.14	.32
19	50	Cauliflower	.60	.30
20	60	Parsnip	.50	.30

Biotin

Background Biotin is found in most foods. It is also made by bacteria that live in our intestines.

Importance Biotin is necessary for maintaining healthy skin, hair, sweat glands, nerves and bone marrow. Like other B-group vitamins, it plays a part in the metabolism of carbohydrates, proteins and (particularly) fats. It is used by some practitioners in the treatment of problems of the scalp and skin (including dandruff and hair loss).

Deficiency Since it is widely available in the diet, biotin deficiency is rare. In cases of extremely poor nutrition, however, it may cause dry, scaly skin, hair loss, fatigue, nausea and loss of appetite as well as muscle pains, pins and needles, anaemia and a raised blood cholesterol level.

Toxicity Biotin is thought to be non-toxic.

20 good sources of Biotin found in common plant foods

	Portion size (g)	Type	µg per 100g	µg per portion
1	90	Tempeh	53.00	47.70
2	90	Soya beans, boiled	25.00	22.50
3	20	Peanut butter	102.00	20.40
4	15	Hazelnuts	76.00	11.40
5	15	Peanuts	72.00	10.80
6	15	Almonds	64.00	9.60
7	50	Muesli	15.00	7.50
8	90	Black-eyed beans, boiled	7.00	6.30
9	50	Mushrooms	12.00	6.00
10	145	Avocado	3.60	5.22
11	90	Mange tout peas	5.30	4.77
12	135	Baked beans	2.50	3.38
13	7	Wheat bran	45.00	3.15
14	120	Banana	2.60	3.12
15	15	Oatmeal	20.00	3.00
16	15	Walnuts	19.00	2.85
17	90	Broad beans	2.70	2.43
18	20	Tahini paste	11.00	2.20
19	50	Globe artichoke	4.10	2.05
20	75	Redcurrants	2.60	1.95

Water soluble vitamins – vitamin C

Vitamin C

Background Vitamin C is found in all fresh fruits and vegetables. Meat and cereals contain negligible amounts. Since vitamin C is soluble in water, the vitamin C content of vegetables and fruits is reduced by cooking them in water.

Importance Vitamin C is necessary for maintaining the health of all body tissues. It is an important anti-oxidant, and is necessary for the proper absorption and use of iron. Vitamin C plays a vital role in wound healing and appears to be necessary for the efficient functioning of our immune system. Its possible effects on allergy, blood fat levels and cancer are the subject of much debate, so far unresolved.

Deficiency Chronic vitamin C deficiency causes scurvy, a condition much feared by seafarers of old, who lived mainly on a diet of meat and biscuits. The Scottish physician, James Lind, showed in 1772 that including some citrus fruit in the diet could both cure and prevent scurvy.

Nowadays, vitamin C deficiency is only seen in cases of severe malnutrition, malabsorption or chronic alcoholism. The symptoms are bruising, bleeding gums, slow healing wounds and, in severe cases, swollen, painful joints. Smokers, cancer sufferers and people with rheumatoid arthritis all have decreased amounts of vitamin C in their blood.

Toxicity There is much debate about the wisdom of taking very large amounts of vitamin C each day. More than 2 or 3 grams is likely to produce diarrhoea, and may increase the risk of developing kidney stones. High-doses of vitamin C also interfere with the accuracy of dipsticks used by diabetics to check urine sugar levels.

20 good sources of vitamin C found in common plant foods

	Portion size (g)	Type	mg per 100g	mg per portion
1	120	Guava	230	276
2	120	Red pepper	140	168
3	90	Spring greens	180	162
4	75	Blackcurrants	200	150
5	120	Green pepper	120	144
6	90	Brussels sprouts	115	104
7	90	Curly kale	110	99
8	120	Pawpaw	60	72
9	75	Strawberries	77	58
10	50	Purple broccoli	110	55
11	90	Mange tout peas	54	49
12	80	Lemon	58	46
13	120	Mango	37	44
14	90	Cabbage	49	44
15	50	Broccoli	87	44
16	80	Clementines	54	43
17	80	Oranges	54	43
18	100	Nectarines	37	37
19	60	Kiwi	59	35
20	100	Peaches	31	31

Fat-soluble vitamins

Vitamin A (Beta-carotene and retinol)

Background   Vitamin A occurs in plants in the form of yellow and orange pigments called carotenes. The most important carotene, beta-carotene, is found in yellow and orange fruits and vegetables, and also in green leaves. Animal-derived vitamin A, retinol, is produced from beta-carotene eaten in the diet and is stored in the liver. About one sixth of the beta-carotene eaten is turned into retinol.

Importance   Beta-carotene is an important anti-oxidant vitamin. Retinol is essential for normal vision and for healthy skin and other tissues.

Deficiency   Vitamin A deficiency is rare, but can be caused by intestinal disease. Retinol deficiency leads to night-blindness, and is still a major cause of eye disease and blindness (xeropthalmia) amongst grossly malnourished children under the age of four in very poor parts of the world. Breast feeding provides the best protection against childhood xeropthalmia.

Toxicity   Too much retinol (more than 9000 micrograms per day) can cause bone and liver damage. Pregnant women should not eat more than 3000 micrograms of retinol per day, since higher amounts may harm the developing baby. (Lamb, ox, chicken, calf and pig liver all contain between 5000 and 11,000 micrograms of retinol per portion.) Beta-carotene from plants is completely non-toxic, although very large amounts may cause yellow discoloration of the skin. It can provide the body with all the vitamin A it needs for health.

20 good sources of Vitamin A found in common plant foods

Portion size (g)	Type	Beta-car. µg per 100g	Beta-car. µg per portion	µg Retinol equiv.
1	130	Sweet potato	5140	6682	1114
2	60	Carrot	8115	4869	812
3	120	Red pepper	3840	4608	768
4	120	Butternut squash	3630	4356	726
5	90	Swiss chard	4625	4163	694
6	90	Spinach	3535	3182	530
7	90	Curly kale	3145	2831	472
8	90	Spring greens	2630	2367	395
9	120	Mango	1800	2160	360

table continues

	Portion size (g)	Type	Beta-car. µg per 100g	Beta-car. µg per portion	µg Retinol equiv.
10	175	Cantaloupe melon	1000	1750	292
11	3	Paprika	36250	1088	181
12	120	Pawpaw	810	972	162
13	100	Sharon fruit	950	950	158
14	90	Savoy cabbage	995	896	149
15	120	Tomato	640	768	128
16	120	Courgette	610	732	122
17	90	Mange tout peas	695	626	104
18	120	Pumpkin	450	540	90
19	50	Butterhead lettuce	910	455	76
20	60	Leek	735	441	74

Vitamin D

Background   Although vitamin D is added to a number of fortified foods (such as margarines and breakfast cereals), only a few foods (eg. eggs, butter and oily fish) contain vitamin D naturally. However, vitamin D in food is not necessary for most people (even babies), since we all produce vitamin D internally by the action of sunlight on our skin. Even skyshine on a cloudy day causes vitamin D production. The best way to ensure adequate vitamin D is to spend some time each day in the open air.

Importance   Vitamin D is necessary to help us absorb calcium from our food, and a deficiency can lead to softening of the bones and deformity (known as rickets in children and osteomalacia in adults).

Deficiency   Generally speaking, vitamin D deficiency is rare. However, black people and Asian vegetarians living in countries where climate restricts exposure to daylight seem to be slightly more at risk of vitamin D deficiency than Caucasians, and there is also some evidence that babies on breast milk alone after four to six months of age may need some extra dietary vitamin D to ensure proper nourishment. Elderly people who are housebound also need to ensure an adequate vitamin D intake in their diet. There is no evidence that an animal-produce-free diet increases the risk of vitamin D deficiency, as long as it provides sufficient calories and the right amount of protein – and as long as there is regular exposure to daylight. Fortified foods (margarines, plant milks, etc.) containing added plant vitamin D2 (ergocalciferol) can, of course, be used as extra insurance, where necessary.

Toxicity Too much vitamin D (only usually seen in cases where an excessive dose of Vitamin D has been used to treat rickets or osteomalacia) is toxic, and causes an abnormally high blood calcium level. This may produce a variety of problems, including kidney damage.

Vitamin E

Background Vitamin E is a fat-soluble vitamin found in a wide variety of foods.

Importance Vitamin E is an important anti-oxidant, and may also have a role in maintaining the normal function of red blood cells.

Deficiency Being fat-soluble, vitamin E is easily stored in the body. This, combined with its wide availability in food, makes deficiency (which may cause muscle, nerve and liver damage) extremely rare. However, there is some evidence that anti-oxidants such as vitamin E have a role in preventing the development of bowel cancer, breast cancer and coronary heart disease; it may be that the amount of vitamin E necessary to avoid any obvious deficiency is less than the amount required to gain its disease-preventing benefits.

Smokers in particular should be aware of the importance of vitamin E in the diet, as tobacco smoke contains large amounts of free radicals.

Toxicity When obtained from food, vitamin E has no toxic effects. Very high doses of vitamin E supplements have been reported to cause breast soreness, muscle weakness, psychological disturbance and gastro-intestinal upset in some people, and may possibly affect thyroid function.

18 good sources of Vitamin E found in common plant foods

	Portion size (g)	Type	mg per 100g	mg per portion
1	15	Wheatgerm oil	136.70	20.51
2	40	Sundried tomatoes	23.98	9.59
3	130	Sweet potato	5.96	7.75
4	15	Sunflower oil	49.20	7.38
5	15	Safflower oil	40.70	6.11
6	15	Sunflower seeds	37.77	5.67
7	145	Avocado	3.20	4.64
8	15	Hazelnuts	24.98	3.75
9	15	Almonds	23.96	3.59

table continues

	Portion size (g)	Type	mg per 100g	mg per portion
10	15	Corn oil	17.20	2.58
11	7	Polyunsaturated margarine	32.60	2.28
12	120	Butternut squash	1.83	2.20
13	15	Pine nuts	13.65	2.05
14	75	Blackberries	2.37	1.78
15	50	Muesli	3.20	1.60
16	90	Spinach	1.71	1.54
17	90	Curly kale	1.70	1.53
18	15	Peanuts	10.09	1.51

Vitamin K

Background   Vitamin K in nature is produced by plants (vitamin K1) and by bacteria (vitamin K2). Most of the vitamin K in the human diet comes from green leafy vegetables, but bacteria in our intestines also contribute significantly to our vitamin K levels, especially if our diet is high in non-starch polysaccharides (fibre). The body stores vitamin K in the liver and recycles vitamin K molecules many times before breaking down and excreting them.

Importance   Vitamin K is known as the coagulation vitamin, and is a vital component of our blood clotting system. It has also been suggested that it may have a role in the prevention of osteoporosis.

Deficiency   Since vitamin K is widely available in plant-based foods, is made by gut bacteria and is stored in the liver, cases of deficiency are rare. However, diseases that affect the absorption of fat from our diet (vitamin K is fat-soluble, remember), such as coeliac disease, pancreatitis, cystic fibrosis and chronic liver disease, may produce various problems associated with poor blood clotting – easy bruising and bleeding, for example. Some antibiotics also reduce our vitamin K intake by destroying normal vitamin K-producing gut bacteria.

A small number of newborn babies suffer from haemorrhagic disease of the newborn (HDN) which is apparently related to a deficiency of vitamin K. Use of vitamin K injections soon after birth is not now recommended since there is some evidence that this practice increases the risk of childhood cancer. The current orthodox view is that mothers should be given some extra vitamin K in the few days before birth, and that the newborn should receive its protective dose of vitamin K by mouth. The true value of this intervention in reducing the risk of HDN is not known.

Toxicity   Natural vitamin K is harmless, even when eaten in large amounts.

Good food sources   Precise data on the vitamin K content of common foods is not available. However, broccoli, spinach, parsley, cabbage (particularly the outer leaves), curly kale, spring greens, cauliflower and peas all contain high levels of vitamin K. Soya based margarines and vegetable oils are also good sources (but only when reasonably fresh since vitamin K is destroyed by exposure to light).

MINERALS

Understanding of how minerals are used by the body is still developing, but in general terms it is known that they perform four functions:

1. They help to build and maintain teeth and bones.
2. They play a part in controlling the amount and composition of body fluids.
3. They allow vitamins to function properly.
4. They work with enzymes and other chemicals involved in metabolism.

All the minerals essential to health can be obtained from food. Some – the major minerals – are needed in large quantities, but others – the trace elements – are only required in tiny amounts. The importance of trace elements has only been recognized in recent years.

A few minerals (eg. sodium, potassium and chloride) are absorbed completely from the food we eat, but the majority pass through the gut with only about ten to fifteen percent being absorbed (the precise amount depending on the body's needs at the time).

Because of this, it is often wasteful to take minerals in high dosages for their therapeutic effects, because the body won't absorb what it doesn't need. Some unabsorbed minerals can even cause digestive problems. For example, iron, when taken in excess can cause stomach pain, colic and constipation. It is usually best to get the minerals we need from our food, because minerals in food are made available in a gradual, easy to absorb way during digestion, and come ready packaged with other nutrients that assist absorption. Parsley, for example, contains plenty of iron but also plenty of vitamin C, which helps the iron to be absorbed.

Bear in mind that all minerals – major and trace elements – come from the earth via soil and water. Whether we eat them directly in plant foods or indirectly in animal foods, any mineral deficiency in the soil is likely to be reflected in food.

Major Minerals

Calcium

Background Calcium is found in many different foods and sometimes (in hard water areas) in drinking water. Only about twenty to thirty percent of any calcium eaten is actually absorbed, however. Calcium absorption depends on the presence of vitamin D (see Chapter Eight and Appendix Two).

Importance Calcium gives structure and strength to teeth and bones, which between them contain ninety-nine percent of all calcium in the body. The remaining one percent plays a vital role in maintaining the healthy function of muscles (including the heart), nerves, enzymes and hormones, and a variety of mechanisms operate to ensure that enough non-bone calcium is always available to the body. The bones and teeth act as a sort of calcium bank, with calcium constantly being withdrawn and deposited according to need.

Deficiency If there is not enough calcium in the diet, overdrawing from the calcium bank may produce a variety of conditions, including softening of the bones (osteomalacia and rickets) and tooth decay. Some people also link osteoporosis with long-standing nutritional calcium deficiency, but a direct link between low dietary calcium and osteoporosis has not been established (see Chapter Eight). High-protein diets cause calcium to be lost from the body in the urine.

In the past, calcium was added to all British flours because it was thought that phytates in grains interfered with calcium absorption. The current expert view is that this effect is not significant, and thus that fortification of flour with calcium is not necessary.

Toxicity Too much dietary calcium – from nutritional supplements or (more commonly) from long-term taking of calcium-containing indigestion tablets – can cause a variety of problems including nausea, depression and kidney damage.

20 good sources of Calcium found in common plant foods

	Portion size (g)	Type	mg per 100g	mg per portion
1	90	Tofu, fried	1480	1332
2	90	Tofu, steamed	510	459
3	120	Okra	160	192

table continues

	Portion size (g)	Type	mg per 100g	mg per portion
4	90	Spring greens	210	189
5	90	Spinach	170	153
6	20	Tahini paste	680	136
7	140	Stewed rhubarb	93	130
8	90	Curly kale	130	117
9	90	Tempeh	120	108
10	15	Sesame seeds	670	101
11	50	Purple sprouting broccoli	200	100
12	60	Spring onions	140	84
13	30	Dried figs	250	75
14	90	Soya beans	83	75
15	20	Carob flour	350	70
16	20	Self-raising flour	350	70
17	80	Lemon	85	68
18	50	Muesli	120	60
19	90	Haricot beans, boiled	65	59
20	3	Celery seeds	1770	53

Note

Human milk contains 34mg/100g, cow's milk contains 120mg/100g, eggs 52mg/100g and cheese 800mg/100g.

Magnesium

Background Magnesium is the second most abundant mineral in the body after calcium. About seventy percent of it is found in the bones and teeth; the rest is inside cells. It is abundant in food, especially in vegetables, and it is an essential component of the green plant pigment chlorophyll. Less than half the magnesium we eat is absorbed.

Importance Magnesium plays an essential part in the enzyme systems that help us to make use of the energy stored in our tissues. It is also needed to enable vitamin B1 and vitamin B6 to work efficiently. Magnesium helps the body to absorb and retain calcium, and deposit it in the bones.

Deficiency Magnesium deficiency may occur as a result of severe diarrhoea, alcoholism, diabetes and taking diuretics. Diets high in refined and processed foods are also linked with magnesium deficiency. Excess calcium in the diet suppresses magnesium absorption.

Some practitioners believe that magnesium deficiency is a factor in epilepsy, heart disease, high blood pressure, pre-menstrual syndrome, osteoporosis and mental disturbance. Severe magnesium deficiency causes muscle cramps and convulsions.

Toxicity High doses of magnesium tend to pass through the gut without being absorbed. As a result, they may cause diarrhoea. Magnesium toxicity is rare, and usually only seen in people with kidney failure. The effects are thirst, flushing and low blood pressure followed by unconsciousness, heart failure and death.

20 good sources of Magnesium found in common plant foods

	Portion size (g)	Type	mg per 100g	mg per portion
1	15	Brazil nuts	590.0	88.5
2	120	Okra	71.0	85.2
3	15	Melon seeds	510.0	76.5
4	20	Tahini paste	380.0	76.0
5	90	Swiss chard	81.0	72.9
6	150	Brown rice	43.0	64.5
7	90	Tempeh	70.0	63.0
8	15	Sunflower seeds	390.0	58.5
9	90	Soya beans	63.0	56.7
10	15	Sesame seeds	370.0	55.5
11	90	Aduki and pinto beans (average)	58.0	52.2
12	90	Spinach	54.0	48.6
13	90	Black-eyed beans	52.0	46.8
14	125	Sweetcorn-on-the-cob	37.0	46.3
15	50	Muesli	85.0	42.5
16	120	Bananas	34.0	40.8
17	120	Butternut squash	34.0	40.8
18	15	Almonds, cashews, pine nuts and pumpkin seeds	270.0	40.5
19	120	Acorn squash	32.0	38.4
20	7	Wheat bran	520.0	36.4

Phosphorus

Background Phosphorus is abundant in the body, and eighty five percent of it is found in the bones and teeth. The rest is inside cells. It is a component of nearly all foodstuffs.

Importance Phosphorus, as part of a chemical known as ATP, plays a vital role in the release and use of energy from food. It is also an important building block for various proteins, carbohydrates and fats.

Deficiency Low blood levels of phosphorus may be caused by alcoholism, some drugs, vitamin D deficiency and pregnancy. Blood phosphorus levels also decrease when the body is subjected to severe injury. Phosphorus deficiency may lead to softening of the bones (osteomalacia), muscle weakness and impaired immunity. In children it produces poor growth. However, phosphorus deficiency is very rare.

Babies require a correct balance between calcium and phosphorus in their milk because too much phosphorus (for example, from cow's milk not processed into suitable infant formulae) will cause muscle spasms.

Toxicity Too much phosphorus in the diet upsets the balance between calcium and phosphorus in the body. The maximum daily intake should be less than 70 milligrams per kilo of body weight (a maximum of 4900 milligrams for a 70 kilogram person).

20 good sources of Phosphorus found in common plant foods

	Portion size (g)	Type	mg per 100g	mg per portion
1	4	Baking powder	8430	337
2	150	Brown rice, cooked	120	180
3	90	Tempeh	200	180
4	20	Tahini paste	730	146
5	50	Muesli	280	140
6	20	Soya flour	600	120
7	90	Peas, raw	130	117
8	90	Beans and lentils (average)	128	115
9	15	Nuts and seeds (average)	682	102
10	125	Sweetcorn	81	101
11	20	Self-raising flour	450	90
12	90	Tofu	95	86
13	130	Sweet potato	65	85
14	7	Wheat bran	1200	84
15	90	Spring greens	91	82
16	150	White rice, cooked	54	81
17	20	Pearl barley	380	76
18	20	Rye flour	360	72
19	120	Okra	59	71
20	90	Brussels sprouts	77	69

Potassium

Background   A plant-based diet consisting mainly of unadulterated fresh foods will contain more potassium than sodium. A 'normal' Western diet – based largely on processed foods of animal origin – contains more sodium than potassium. It has been suggested that potassium/sodium imbalance may play a part in a number of the diseases common in our society, including high blood pressure.

Importance   Potassium is found in all body cells; our hearts, muscles and nerves could not function without it. So the body controls its potassium levels very carefully, maintaining a fine balance between the amount of potassium inside cells and the amount of sodium (and chloride) outside cells. Potassium is also involved in maintaining normal blood sugar levels.

Deficiency   Potassium deficiency can be caused by a variety of gastro-intestinal disorders, particularly those involving chronic diarrhoea and malabsorption. It is also a feature of severe diabetes, and a side-effect of certain drugs (including diuretics, steroids and laxatives). Too much salt in the diet tends to reduce the amount of potassium in the body.

Features of potassium deficiency include muscle weakness and cramps, poor appetite, tiredness, depression, constipation and palpitations. Severe deficiency may even lead to heart failure.

Toxicity   Potassium excess can be caused by severe dehydration, kidney failure and adrenal gland failure; in severe cases it produces cardiac arrest. Extremely high intakes of potassium by mouth (eg. 18 grams or more per day in the form of supplements) are also toxic.

20 good sources of Potassium found in common plant foods

	Portion size (g)	Type	mg per 100 g	mg per portion
1	145	Avocado	450	653
2	180	Potatoes	360	648
3	130	Sweet potato	480	624
4	30	Dried apricots	1880	564
5	120	Acorn squash	440	528
6	90	Aduki beans	570	513
7	120	Banana	400	480
8	90	Pigeon peas	510	459
9	90	Soya beans	510	459

table continues

	Portion size (g)	Type	mg per 100 g	mg per portion
10	90	Spinach	500	450
11	120	Courgette	360	432
12	90	Pinto beans	460	414
13	90	Brussels sprouts	450	405
14	90	Curly kale	450	405
15	120	Okra	330	396
16	90	Butter beans	400	360
17	90	Endive	380	342
18	90	Swiss chard	380	342
19	90	Spring greens	370	333
20	90	Tempeh	370	333

Sodium and Chloride (common salt)

Background The role of salt in the diet is discussed in some detail in Chapter Eight. It occurs naturally in all foodstuffs and has been highly prized as a condiment for centuries.

Importance Sodium and chloride are found in all cells and body fluids, including the blood. They are important in maintaining the correct amount of water in the body, and sodium plays a vital role in both nerve and muscle function.

Deficiency The condition commonly referred to as dehydration is usually the result of a combined loss of water, sodium and chloride. This may happen for a variety of reasons, including severe vomiting or diarrhoea, kidney damage, diuretic therapy, excessive sweating in extreme environments (very hot climate, vigorous exercise, sauna baths, etc.) and burns. The effects of dehydration are exhaustion, nausea and dizziness leading to vomiting and muscle cramps and, in extreme cases, life-threatening shock.

Toxicity Excessive salt intake is clearly linked to the development of high blood pressure and an increased risk of heart disease. The average adult Westerner consumes at least twice as much salt as is actually necessary for health, mostly because of a taste for processed and animal-based food products. This situation is made worse by the fact that, although our salt needs could be easily covered by the natural salt in our food, our habitual desire for salt leads many of us to add large amounts of salt to what we eat. As discussed in Chapter Eight, the easy way to reduce daily salt intake is to increase the amount of unprocessed plant-based foods in our diet and decrease the amount of animal-based or processed foods. The effect of this change is likely to be far more significant than any reduction in the amount of salt added to food.

Sodium (representing salt) content of 20 common plant foods

	Portion size (g)	Type	mg per 100g	mg per portion
1	200	Porridge[1]	560	1120
2	15	Soy sauce	7120	1068
3	135	Baked beans	550	743
4	30	Olives	2250	675
5	50	Hummus	670	335
6	10	Vine leaves	2210	221
7	50	Muesli	380	190
8	90	Swiss chard	210	189
9	30	Rye bread	580	174
10	4	Yeast extract	4300	172
11	30	Wholemeal bread	550	165
12	5	Wakame seaweed	3220	161
13	30	White bread	520	156
14	90	Spinach	140	126
15	15	Roasted peanuts	790	119
16	5	Kombu seaweed	1830	92
17	15	Pistachio nuts, roasted	530	80
18	20	Self-raising flour	360	72
19	20	Peanut butter	350	70
20	60	Celeriac	91	55

[1] Made with water, salt added.

Sulphur

Background The role of sulphur in the human body is not well understood. It forms a part of some proteins (as a part of the amino acids methionine and cystine), and is also a component of two of the B vitamins, thiamin and biotin. Sulphur is found mainly in foods that contain a lot of protein.

Trace elements

Iron

Background Despite the importance of iron to health, the average human body contains only about 3 or 4 grams of it in total. Of this, about sixty percent is found in red blood cells (in the oxygen-carrying chemical haemoglobin), about ten percent in muscles, and about five percent in the blood and in various enzymes. The rest is found in the liver which acts as an iron reserve store for the body.

Iron in food comes in two forms, haem and non-haem. About forty percent of the iron found in animal-based foods is in the haem form. All the iron contained in plant-based foods is in the non-haem form. Haem iron is better absorbed from the gut than non-haem iron, but vitamin C, citric acid and other substances widely found in plant foods greatly increase non-haem iron absorption. In any case, we only absorb between five and fifteen percent of the iron we eat on average, but we do have the capacity to increase our iron absorption in times of need – such as childhood and pregnancy – and when we have lost blood due to injury or surgery.

Importance   Because it is involved with carrying oxygen from our lungs to our tissues (in haemoglobin), iron is one of the most important minerals in the body. Iron containing enzymes enable our cells to release energy from food, our brains to function properly and our livers to detoxify harmful substances. They are involved in the production of certain hormones and also in the manufacture of bile. The iron containing chemical myoglobin provides muscles with a ready reserve of oxygen.

Deficiency   A number of things can interfere with the absorption of iron from food – for example, too much tea, too much soya, too much fibre, too much spinach, too much milk and too many calcium supplements. However, except in cases of obvious malnourishment, particular dietary preferences do not usually cause iron deficiency because nearly all diets (vegetarian and non-vegetarian) contain such a wide variety of foods rich in iron. The body also appears to have a sophisticated ability to look after its iron needs, whatever sorts of food it is presented with.

The main cause of iron deficiency in the West is blood loss – internally or externally – resulting from illness (eg. stomach ulcers, fibroids and haemorrhoids). Heavy periods, excess demand for iron during breast feeding, and very poor quality diets low in vitamin C (and other essential nutrients such as copper), may also lead to iron deficiency. Babies fed on cow's milk risk iron deficiency because cow's milk is low in iron and contains calcium in a form that seriously inhibits iron absorption.

The main symptoms of iron deficiency are persistent tiredness and a tendency to get unusually out of breath after minimal physical exertion. Palpitations, dizziness, headaches and poor concentration may also occur. (Note that healthy women do *not* need to increase their iron intake during pregnancy. The natural lowering of haemoglobin levels that occurs helps to avoid the possibility of premature and low birth-weight babies.)

Toxicity Taking oral iron supplements causes stomach pain and constipation in up to twenty percent of people. High doses of iron are toxic for children, and a single dose of 100g can be lethal for adults.

Too much iron in the body overall leads to iron being deposited abnormally in the tissues – known as iron overload. This can be caused by large blood transfusions and by iron injections given in excess. It may also result from drinking too much cheap wine over many years. Various diseases, including blood and liver disorders, and an hereditary disease called haemochromatosis, cause serious iron overload; this may lead to liver damage, diabetes, heart failure, palpitations, loss of libido, stomach pain, arthritis and liver cancer.

20 good sources of Iron found in common plant foods

	Portion size (g)	Type	mg per 100g	mg per portion
1	90	Tempeh	3.6	3.2
2	90	Lentils	3.5	3.2
3	180	New potatoes (with skin)	1.6	2.9
4	50	Muesli	5.6	2.8
5	90	Spring greens	3.0	2.7
6	90	Endive	2.8	2.5
7	90	Peas	2.8	2.5
8	20	Tahini paste	10.6	2.1
9	3	Cumin seeds	69.0	2.1
10	30	Dried peaches	6.8	2.0
11	90	Chick-peas	2.1	1.9
12	90	Spinach	2.1	1.9
13	90	Beans, average	2.1	1.9
14	90	Swiss chard	1.8	1.6
15	15	Sesame seeds	10.4	1.6
16	90	Curly kale	1.7	1.5
17	15	Pumpkin seeds	10.0	1.5
18	3	Celery seeds	44.9	1.3
19	120	Okra	1.1	1.3
20	30	Dried figs	4.2	1.3

Zinc

Background Zinc is present in variable amounts in many types of food. The body is able to adjust the amount absorbed according to need, but in a typical Western diet, only about thirty percent of the zinc eaten in food is absorbed.

Importance Zinc is used in many different ways by the body. It plays a part in making proteins, breaking down carbohydrates and alcohol, healing wounds, transporting vitamin A, transporting carbon dioxide, making insulin, making prostatic secretions and eliminating waste products from working muscles. There have been suggestions that zinc can be used to treat skin complaints, high blood fat, prostate problems, eating disorders, hyperactivity in children and schizophrenia.

Deficiency The amount of zinc absorbed from food is sensitive to many different factors. Vitamin B6, for example, increases zinc absorption, but taking calcium supplements may reduce it. The high fat/high sugar/high refined food diet common in the West tends to produce a low intake of zinc, and polyphosphate and EDTA food additives can make zinc virtually unabsorbable. Boiling and canning foods also reduces their zinc content.

Alcohol, and some diuretic drugs, cause zinc to be lost from the body in the urine. Surgery, burns, severe weight loss and a number of diseases (including Crohn's disease) can all produce zinc deficiency. Whilst severe zinc deficiency is known to cause a variety of problems including loss of appetite, skin problems, susceptibility to infections, slow healing wounds, hair loss, loss of sense of smell and taste, diarrhoea, apathy, fatigue, white spots on the nails and even psychiatric disturbances, the effects and importance of mild zinc deficiency are not well understood. Mild zinc deficiency is known to cause poor growth in male infants, however; and older children lacking zinc in their diet may develop a habit of eating dirt.

Toxicity Large amounts of zinc (2 grams or more) taken in food supplements produce nausea and vomiting. High doses taken over long periods can also inhibit the absorption of other minerals (including copper, iron and calcium) from the diet. There have been a few cases of zinc poisoning caused by drinking fizzy acidic drinks from zinc-galvanized cans.

20 good sources of Zinc found in common plant foods

	Portion size (g)	Type	mg per 100g	mg per portion
1	90	Aduki beans	2.3	2.1
2	90	Tofu, fried	2.0	1.8
3	90	Tempeh	1.8	1.6
4	90	Lentils	1.4	1.3
5	50	Muesli	2.5	1.3
6	230	Pasta	.5	1.2
7	7	Wheat bran	16.2	1.1
8	90	Chick-peas	1.2	1.1
9	20	Tahini paste	5.4	1.1
10	150	Brown rice	.7	1.1
11	90	Black-eyed beans	1.1	1.0
12	15	Pumpkin seeds	6.6	1.0
13	15	Pine nuts	6.5	1.0
14	50	Irish moss seaweed	1.9	1.0
15	90	Haricot beans	1.0	.9
16	90	Peas	1.0	.9
17	15	Cashew nuts	5.9	.9
18	5	Wheat germ	17.0	.9
19	200	Porridge	.4	.8
20	15	Pecan nuts	5.3	.8

Manganese

Background   Manganese is abundant in vegetables and is also found in high quantities in tea. In the body, manganese is found in bone and as a component of a variety of important enzymes. Absorption from the diet is regulated by the body's needs but, on average, only about ten percent of any manganese eaten is absorbed. If the diet is particularly low in manganese, the mineral is conserved in the body by reducing the rate at which it is lost from the body in the urine.

Importance   Manganese is necessary for proper bone development, efficient protein and fat metabolism, and the production of cholesterol.

Deficiency   Calcium, phosphorus, zinc and cobalt can all inhibit manganese absorption, but clear cases of manganese deficiency are very rare. Lack of manganese has nevertheless been associated with diabetes, heart disease, schizophrenia, epilepsy, cancer, atherosclerosis, myasthenia gravis and rheumatoid arthritis.

Toxicity High intakes of manganese may cause nerve and brain problems resembling Parkinson's disease.

20 good sources of Manganese found in common plant foods

	Portion size (g)	Type	mg per 100g	mg per portion
1	230	Wholemeal spaghetti	.9	2.07
2	50	Oyster mushrooms	3.6	1.80
3	150	Brown rice	.9	1.35
4	50	Muesli	2.6	1.30
5	90	Tempeh	1.4	1.26
6	15	Pine nuts	7.9	1.19
7	90	Tofu, fried	1.2	1.08
8	75	Blackberries	1.4	1.05
9	200	Porridge	.5	.92
10	3	Dried, ground ginger	28.0	.84
11	15	Macadamia nuts	5.5	.83
12	15	Hazelnuts	4.9	.74
13	90	Aduki beans	.8	.72
14	120	Bananas	.6	.72
15	90	Curly kale	.8	.72
16	15	Pecan nuts	4.6	.69
17	75	Mulberries	.9	.68
18	130	Sweet potato	.5	.65
19	7	Wheat bran	9.0	.63
20	90	Chick-peas	.7	.63

Copper

Background Copper is found in various foodstuffs including cereals, nuts, peas, beans, shellfish and liver. In the body it is found in muscles, the liver, bones and the blood. Some intra-uterine contraceptive devices (IUDs) are based on copper, and the mineral has a long-standing reputation for easing the symptoms of arthritis (copper bracelets, etc.).

Importance Copper is involved in the making of red blood cells, in the production of bone and in general body tissue maintenance. It is also necessary for the production of various important chemicals in the nervous system.

Deficiency Copper deficiency is uncommon, but may be caused by malnutrition, malabsorption and chronic diarrhoea. It can also be produced by taking large amounts of zinc, cadmium, fluoride or molybdenum, and by the use of chelating agents (chemicals used to remove toxic minerals from the body). Babies fed entirely on cow's milk over a long period of time may also become copper deficient, because cow's milk contains very little copper.

Copper deficiency is associated with anaemia, osteoporosis, susceptibility to infection and de-pigmentation of the skin and hair. In babies it produces poor growth. Copper deficiency may also be a cause of underactive thyroid.

Toxicity Excess copper is poisonous, and causes nausea, stomach pain, diarrhoea, muscle pains, mood swings, blood disorders and skin problems. High blood levels of copper have been noticed in women on the pill, and in people suffering from zinc deficiency, schizophrenia, epilepsy, rheumatoid arthritis and heart disease. They also occur in people living in areas where the drinking water contains a lot of copper. Foods containing vitamin C, zinc, magnesium and rutin are known to help reduce high levels of copper in the blood.

20 good sources of Copper found in common plant foods

	Portion size (g)	Type	mg per 100g	mg per portion
1	90	Tempeh	.67	.60
2	20	Soya flour	2.92	.58
3	150	White rice	.37	.56
4	150	Brown rice	.33	.50
5	90	Aduki beans	.51	.46
6	90	Pigeon peas	.46	.41
7	50	Mushrooms	.72	.36
8	15	Melon seeds	2.39	.36
9	15	Sunflower seeds	2.27	.34
10	15	Cashew nuts	2.11	.32
11	90	Dal	.34	.31
12	20	Tahini paste	1.48	.30
13	90	Soya beans	.32	.29
14	15	Brazil nuts	1.76	.26
15	90	Chick-peas	.28	.25
16	30	Currants	.81	.24
17	15	Pumpkin seeds	1.57	.24
18	30	Dried pineapple	.74	.22

table continues

	Portion size (g)	Type	mg per 100g	mg per portion
19	15	Sesame seeds	1.46	.22
20	15	Walnuts	1.34	.20

Iodine

Background   The most reliable sources of iodine in the diet come from the sea – fish and seaweeds are extremely rich in iodine. Iodine is routinely added to livestock feed, and so finds its way into milk, making milk a major source of iodine for many people. Sea salt and iodized salt are also important sources of iodine. The amount of iodine in plants varies depending on iodine levels in the soil. Most of the iodine in the body is found in the thyroid gland.

Importance   Iodine is an essential component of the thyroid hormones, which influence nearly all biochemical reactions in the body, and which are necessary for normal growth and physical and mental development.

Deficiency   Iodine deficiency is rare in the West these days, but is still an important health problem in the Third World. It may cause goitre (enlarged thyroid gland) and underactive thyroid (resulting in weight gain, loss of energy, constipation, dry skin and hair and, possibly, psychiatric disturbance). In children, iodine deficiency can lead to retarded growth and severe mental impairment. Japanese, American and Scandinavian research has linked iodine deficiency to breast cancer.

Toxicity   Excess iodine (more than 1000 micrograms per day) may cause thyroid dysfunction in some people. Radioactive iodine from nuclear accidents can cause thyroid cancer. On the other hand, normal iodine in the diet protects against absorption of radioactive iodine.

Since iodine content in food depends on the way in which it is grown or produced, it is not meaningful to give the top twenty iodine sources. Edible seaweeds do provide a reliable supply of iodine, however.

6 good sources of Iodine found in common plant foods

	Portion size (g)	Type	µg per 100g	µg per portion
		Seaweeds		
1	5	Kombu	440670	22034
2	5	Arame	84140	4207
3	5	Hijiki	42670	2134

table continues

Portion size (g)		Type	mg per 100g	mg per portion
4	5	Wakame	16830	842
5	5	Dulse	5970	299
6	1	Nori	1470	15

Selenium

Background   Although the body absorbs selenium efficiently from food, the amount of selenium in the diet is very variable. The amount of selenium in plants, meats and dairy products depends on how much selenium there is in the soil. Acid rain and intensive agriculture involving the use of artificial fertilizers have reduced the average amount of selenium in food.

Importance   Red blood cells need selenium to function properly and selenium also plays an important role in the body's anti-oxidant systems (see Chapter Eight).

Deficiency   Severe selenium deficiency may cause degenerative heart and joint diseases in young people, but these are only seen where soil selenium levels are particularly low (eg. in parts of China and the Soviet Union). The effects of mild or moderate selenium deficiency (eg. from eating a diet consisting mainly of refined and processed foods) are not well understood. There is some evidence that lack of selenium may be associated with heart disease, stroke, male infertility, eye disease, cot death and cancer.

Toxicity   Dietary selenium excess is unlikely, but may result from supplement overdose. The effects are bad breath, hair loss, an itchy skin rash, brittle nails and, in severe cases, disturbances of the nervous system including paralysis.

To avoid toxicity, the maximum recommended daily intake of selenium for adults is 6µg per kilo body weight per day (which, for a person weighing 65kg, is equivalent to 390µg per day).

20 good sources of Selenium found in common plant foods

Portion size (g)		Type	µg per 100g	µg per portion
1	15	Brazil nuts	1530.0	229.5
2	90	Lentils	40.0	36.0
3	20	Wholemeal flour	53.0	10.6

table continues

	Portion size (g)	Type	µg per 100g	µg per portion
4	30	Wholemeal bread	35.0	10.5
5	230	Pasta	4.0	9.2
6	30	White bread	28.0	8.4
7	20	White flour	42.0	8.4
8	15	Sunflower seeds	49.0	7.4
9	90	Pinto beans	6.0	5.4
10	90	Red kidney beans	6.0	5.4
11	15	Cashew nuts	34.0	5.1
12	50	Mushrooms	9.0	4.5
13	90	Soya beans	5.0	4.5
14	90	Haricot beans	4.0	3.6
15	15	Walnuts	19.0	2.9
16	30	Dried peaches	8.0	2.4
17	30	Raisins	8.0	2.4
18	30	Dried apricots	7.0	2.1
19	20	Buckwheat	9.0	1.8
20	50	Celery	3.0	1.5

Other trace elements

Trace elements are currently the subject of much research. The following are known to play important roles in maintaining the health of the human body and mind, but no dietary reference values have been set for them.

Molybdenum

Approximately eighty percent of the molybdenum we eat in food is absorbed. It forms part of three enzymes that are necessary for the metabolism of fat and some proteins. Deficiency is very rare, but in infants may lead to severe slowing of development, abnormalities of the eyes and nervous system, and impaired protein metabolism. Links have also been suggested between molybdenum deficiency and cancer, impotence and tooth decay. Eating too much molybdenum may disturb copper metabolism.

The best plant sources of molybdenum are pulses, grains, cauliflower and spinach.

Cobalt

Cobalt is a component of vitamin B12. Cobalt deficiency is unknown.

Fluoride

Fluoride is involved with the formation of proper structure in bones and teeth, and low intakes have been linked with tooth decay. Whether fluoride is essential for normal teeth and bones remains unproven, however.

Many Western societies have attempted to head off potential tooth decay by adding fluoride to drinking water. However, too much fluoride can cause a syndrome called fluorosis, consisting of discoloured teeth, bone disease and abnormal joints. Fluoride may also inhibit calcium absorption and interfere with iodine metabolism.

Apart from fluoridated drinking water, tea and seafood contain significant amounts of fluoride.

Chromium

Chromium is thought to be necessary for the normal operation of the process by which the body converts blood sugar into energy. A substance called glucose tolerance factor – consisting of chromium, niacin (vitamin B3) and three amino acids – may be the agent responsible for this conversion. Chromium itself, however, may have a direct action on insulin, the hormone which regulates blood sugar levels.

Chromium deficiency may result from a diet high in refined sugar and processed foods, and may also be caused by severe malnutrition, alcoholism, long-term slimming and diabetes. Deficiency has been linked to high blood fat levels, nervous system disorders and to diabetes that fails to respond properly to insulin treatment.

Chromium is fairly widely distributed in common foods, and is found particularly in the outer layers of vegetables and whole grains. Good sources include potato, green pepper, apple, parsnip, banana, spinach, carrot, wholemeal bread and wheatgerm. All refined and processed foods are low in chromium.

Trace elements are very difficult to study because the mechanisms by which the body absorbs, uses, stores and excretes them are not fully understood. What is more, it is virtually impossible to measure everything that goes in to and comes out of a human body going about its normal business – and especially difficult to measure those substances that are eaten only in tiny amounts.

However, the following trace elements are known to have some role in maintenance of good health:

Strontium   present in bones (not the radioactive form, which is produced in nuclear explosions!)

Aluminium   present in bones. Aluminium excess is known to be toxic, however.

Boron   present in cell membranes.

Lithium   currently used therapeutically to treat manic depressive illness. Makes psoriasis worse.

Arsenic   involved in the metabolism of some amino acids. Used therapeutically in the past – often with disastrous results.

Bromine   used by the body in some circumstances as a substitute for chloride and iodine.

Nickel   involved in the metabolism of some amino acids.

Silicon   provides strength in bone and other tissues.

Vanadium   involved in various metabolic reactions. Deficiency causes neurological, skeletal and thyroid problems.

FURTHER READING

R. Ballentine, *Diet and Nutrition, A Holistic Approach* (Honesdale, Pennsylvania, The Himalayan International Institute, 1982).

M. Bircher-Benner, *Food Science for All*, 2nd edition, edited by A. Eiloart (London, C.W. Daniels Company, 1939).

H.G. Bieler, *Food is Your Best Medicine* (London, Neville Spearman, 1968).

British Herbal Association's Scientific Committee, *British Herbal Pharmacopoeia* (Cowling, West Yorkshire, British Herbal Medicine Association, 1983).

G. Cannon, *The Politics of Food* (London, Century Hutchinson, 1987).

W. Chan, J. Brown and D.H. Buss, *Miscellaneous Foods*, supplement to *McCance and Widdowson's The Composition of Foods* (Cambridge and London, The Royal Society of Chemistry and the Ministry of Agriculture, 1994).

W.H. Cook, *The Physio-Medical Dispensatory* (Portland, Oregon, Eclectic Medical Publications, 1985).

H. Crawley for Ministry of Agriculture, Fisheries and Food, *Food Portion Sizes* (London, Her Majesty's Stationery Office, 1992).

M. Fukuoka, *The One-Straw Revolution* (Rodale Press, USA, 1978).

J.S. Garrow and W.P.T. James, *Human Nutrition and Dietetics*, 9th edition (Edinburgh, Churchill Livingstone, 1993).

M. Grieve, *A Modern Herbal*, edited by C.F. Leyel (London, Tiger Books International, 1992).

B. Griggs, *Green Pharmacy* (London, Jill Norman & Hobhouse, 1981).

D. Hall, *The Book of Herbs* (London, Pan Books, 1976).

M. Hanssen, *E for Additives* (Wellingborough, Northamptonshire, UK, Thorsons, 1984).

R. Hart, *Forest Gardening* (Dartington, Devon, UK, Green Earth Books, 1996).

D. Hoffmann, *The Holistic Herbal* (Forres, Scotland, The Findhorn Press, 1983).

B. Holland, I.D. Unwin and D.H. Buss, *Cereals and Cereal Products*, supplement to *McCance and Widdowson's The Composition of Foods* (Cambridge and London, The Royal Society of Chemistry and the Ministry of Agriculture, 1988).

B. Holland, I.D. Unwin and D.H. Buss, *Fruits and Nuts*, supplement to *McCance and Widdowson's The Composition of Foods* (Cambridge and London, The Royal Society of Chemistry and the Ministry of Agriculture, 1992).

B. Holland, I.D. Unwin and D.H. Buss, *Vegetables, Herbs and Spices*, supplement to *McCance and Widdowson's The Composition of Foods* (Cambridge and London, The Royal Society of Chemistry and the Ministry of Agriculture, 1991).

B. Kew, *The Pocket Book of Animal Facts and Figures* (London, Green Print, 1991).

M. Klaper, *Vegan Nutrition – Pure and Simple* (Umatilla, Florida, Gentle World, 1987).

G.R. Langley, *Vegan Nutrition*, 2nd edition (St Leonards-on-Sea, E. Sussex, UK, The Vegan Society, 1995).

H. Lindlahr, *Natural Therapeutics*, Volume III – Dietetics, edited by J. Proby (Saffron Walden, Essex, UK, C.W. Daniels Company, 1983).

T. Lobstein for The London Food Commision, *Fast Food Facts* (London, Camden Press, 1988).

The London Food Commission, *Food Adulteration and How to Beat it* (London, Unwin Hyman, 1988).

F. Moore Lappé, *Diet for a Small Planet* (New York, Ballantine Books, 1974).

H. Nielsen, *Lægeplanter i Farver* (Copenhagen, Politikens Forlag, 1976).

Parents For Safe Food, *Safe Food Handbook*, edited by Joan and Derek Taylor (London, Ebury Press, 1990).

A.A. Paul and D.A.T. Southgate, *McCance and Widdowson's The Composition of Foods*, 4th edition (London, Her Majesty's Stationery Office, 1978).

A.A. Paul, D.A.T. Southgate and J. Russel, *Amino Acids and Fatty Acids*, supplement to *McCance and Widdowson's The Composition of Foods* (London, Her Majesty's Stationery Office, 1990).

A. Paxton, *The Food Miles Report: the Dangers of Long Distance Food Transport* (London, The Safe Alliance, 1994).

S. Ray, *Indian Vegetarian Cooking* (London, The Apple Press, 1988).

J. Robbins, *Diet for a New America* (Walpole, New Hampshire, Stillpoint Publishing, 1987).

J. Salmon for Department of Health, *Dietary Reference Values – A Guide* (London, Her Majesty's Stationery Office, 1991).

S. Stender, J. Dyerberg, G. Hølmer, L. Ovesen, B. Sandström, *Transfedtsyrernes Betydning for Sundheden* (Copenhagen, Ernæringsrådet, 1995).

A. Wakeman and G. Baskerville, *The Vegan Cookbook* (London, Faber and Faber, 1991).

USEFUL ADDRESSES

The United Kingdom

The Arid Lands Initiative, Machpelah Works, Burnley Road, Hebden Bridge, West Yorkshire HX7 8AU, UK.

The British College of Naturopathy & Osteopathy, Frazer House, 6 Netherhall Gardens, London NW3 5RR, UK

The British Naturopathic Association, Frazer House, 6 Netherhall Gardens, London NW3 5RR, UK.

The British Natural Hygiene Society, Keki Sidhwa, Shalinar, 3 Harold Grove, Frinton-on-Sea, Essex CO13 9BD, UK.

Compassion in World Farming, Charles House, 5a Charles Street, Petersfield, Hants GU32 3EH, UK.

The Ethical Consumer Guide, ECRA Publishing Ltd, 5th Floor, 16 Nicholas St, Manchester M1 4EJ, UK.

The Food Commission, 3rd Floor, 5–11 Worship Street, London EC2A 2BH, UK.

General Council and Register of Naturopaths, Goswell House, 2 Goswell Road, Street, Somerset BA16 0JG, UK.

The Herb Society, 134 Buckingham Palace Road, London SW1W 9SA, UK.

Movement for Compassionate Living, 47 Highlands Road, Leatherhead, Surrey KT22 8NQ, UK.

The National Institute of Medical Herbalists, 56 Longbrook Street, Exeter, Devon EX4 6AH, UK.

Planetary Connections, The Six Bells, Church Street, Bishops Castle, Shropshire SY9 5AA, UK.

SAFE Alliance, 38 Ebury Street, London SW1W 0LU, UK.

The Soil Association, 86–88 Colston Street, Bristol, Avon BS1 5BB, UK.

The United States

American Association of Naturopathic Physicians, PO Box 20386, Seattle, WA 98102, USA.

The American Herb Association, PO Box 1673, Nevada City, CA 95959, USA.

American Naturopathic Medical Association, PO Box 19221, Las Vegas, NV 89132, USA.

Center for Science in the Public Interest/Americans for Safe Food, 1501 16th Street, N.W. Washington DC 20036, USA.

EarthSave Foundation, PO Box 949, Felton, CA 95018–0949, USA.

Humane Farming Association, 1550 California Street, Suite 6, San Francisco, CA 94109, USA.

Natural Hygiene Society, 12816 Race Track Road, Tampa, FL 33625, USA.

The North East Herbal Association, PO Box 479, Milton, NY 12547, USA.

Whole Life, 89 Fifth Avenue, Suite 600, New York, NY 10003, USA.

Canada

Canadian Natural Hygiene Society, PO Box 235, Station T, Toronto, Ontario, M6B 4A1, Canada.

The Ontario Herbalists' Association, 7 Alpine Avenue, Toronto, Ontario, M6P 3R6, Canada.

Ontario Naturopathic Association, 60 Berl Avenue, Toronto, Ontario, M8Y 3C7, Canada.

Australia

The Australian Traditional Medicine Society, PO Box 442, Ryde, 2112, New South Wales, Australia.

The National Herbalists Association of Australia, PO Box 65, Kingsgrove 2208, Australia.

New Zealand

Natural Hygiene Society of Aotearoa/New Zealand, Omanawa, 24 Turere Place, Wanganui, Aotearoa, New Zealand.

South Pacific College of Natural Therapeutics, PO Box 11311, Auckland, New Zealand.

South Africa

School of Health Sciences, Technikon Natal, PO Box 953, Durban 4000, Natal, South Africa.

Israel

Israeli College of Natural Medicine, PO Box 29627, Tel Aviv, 61296, Israel.

INDEX

raisins:
   mint and raisin spread, 181
Ramadan, 130
raw food, 87–8, 91, 124–6
recipes, 149–58
Recommended Daily Amounts (RDAs), 22–3, 24
red lentil soup, 149–50
Reference Nutrient Intakes (RNIs), 23, 24
refined foods, 144
relaxation, 118, 139
religious fasting, 130
relish, horseradish, 173
rest, 118, 139
retinol, 227–8
Reuben, Dr David, 77
Rhazes, 3
rheumatism, 66
riboflavin, 217–18
rice:
   cashew nut paella, 153–4
   catabolic diets, 124–5
   dal with rice, 156–7
   Scottish nettle pudding, 177–8
rickets, 89
roots, 20
   Comparison Charts, 46, 50
   diet diary, 31–2, 37
   minerals and trace elements, 200
   nutritional content, 193
   vitamin content, 207
   Weekly Running Total Chart, 55
rosemary, 182–5
   bath, 184
   incense, 184
   oil, 184–5
   rosemary soup, 184
   rosemary tea, 184
   spaghetti with herb sauce, 183–4
   tonic hair rinse, 185
Rosmarinus officinalis, 182

Safe Intakes, 23
safflower oil, 84
salad dressing, 157–8
salads:
   beetroot, 161
   mint and beetroot, 182
   winter, 157
Salerno, 3
salt, 15, 66–8, 238–9
saturated fats, 10, 80, 82, 83n., 84
sauces:
   almond horseradish, 172
   cold horseradish, 172
   hot horseradish, 173
   mushroom and thyme, 186
Scottish nettle pudding, 177–8
seaweeds, 91

seeds, 21
   Comparison Charts, 46–7, 50–1
   diet diary, 33–4, 37–8
   minerals and trace elements, 202–4
   nutritional content, 195–7
   vitamin content, 209–11
   Weekly Running Total Chart, 56–8
selenium, 86, 87, 247–8
Shaw, George Bernard, 76
sheep's milk, 107
shepherd's pie, 155
Shoerats, Harry, 103–4
silicon, 250
Six-Step Guide, 43–5
Skelton, John, 4
sleep, 114
slimming, 96–100
smoking, 29, 31, 86, 92, 112, 128, 134
snacks:
   anabolic diet, 142
   Comparison Charts, 49, 53
   diet diary, 36, 40
   Weekly Running Total Chart, 61
sodium chloride, 66–8, 238–9
soil, 19
soluble fibre, 69
soups:
   asparagus, 150
   beetroot, 151
   red lentil, 149–50
   rosemary, 184
soya, 91, 94–6
soya milk, 107
spaghetti: spaghetti with herb sauce, 183–4
   spaghetti with spinach and basil sauce, 155–6
spices, 144
   Comparison Charts, 47, 51
   diet diary, 34, 38
   minerals and trace elements, 204
   nutritional content, 197
   vitamin content, 211
   Weekly Running Total Chart, 58
spinach and basil sauce, spaghetti with, 155–6
spirulina, 91
sports, 64
spread, mint and raisin, 181
starchy foods, 88
stems, 20
   Comparison Charts, 46, 50
   diet diary, 32, 37
   minerals and trace elements, 200
   nutritional content, 193
   vitamin content, 207
   Weekly Running Total Chart, 55
steroid hormones, 118
stimulants, 144, 188
strawberries, bananas with, 175
stress, 114–15, 137, 147
strokes, 24–5, 77, 96